Figure Friendly Meals in Minutes

CONCITA THOMAS

DEDICATION

This book is dedicated to everyone who, like me, wants to feed yourself and your family well without spending a lot of time in the kitchen.

ACKNOWLEDGMENTS

The joy that has come from creating this book would not have been possible without my support system. As with anything I do in life, this project has been a team effort.

First, as always, I acknowledge God for placing talent, passion, and purpose inside of me. Thank you for choosing me.

My husband, Al, is my biggest cheerleader and the person who keeps my feet planted even when my head is in the clouds. Thank you for challenging my timeline as well as every suggestion and honest critique. Most of all, thanks for keeping the household running on the days I spent countless hours in the kitchen and at my desk.

My children, AJ and Jackie, are my motivation. Thank you for taste testing my recipes and letting me know when my meals weren't "Kid Approved". Your input is priceless.

My extended family truly is the wind beneath my wings. Thanks for cheering me on even when you don't quite understand what I'm doing.

My Sorors and friends are my trusted confidantes. Thanks for always challenging me to fully step into what I've been called to do in this world.

My business team helps me keep the company moving forward even when I'm laser focused on a specific project. Niambi, thank you for keeping things rolling with my project plans and social media. Julia, thank you for creating the beautiful cover and countless other graphics for the brand. Gynisse, thank you for your gift of telling a story through photography. Our shoots are always so much fun.

My clients give me a place to serve every day. All of this would just be theory without your willingness to put the strategies I create to use. Thank you for your trust.

Table of Contents

Introduction 1

Part I: Guidelines & Strategies 3

Chapter 1: What is a Figure Friendly Meal? 5

Chapter 2: Meals in Minutes Cooking Strategy 11

Part II: The Recipes 25

Chapter 3: Chicken 27

Chapter 4: Ground Meat 51

Chapter 5: Fish & Seafood 73

Chapter 6: Entree Salads 93

Part III: Beyond the Recipes 115

Chapter 7: Spice & Herb Combinations by Cuisine 117

Chapter 8: Grocery & Pantry Staples 121

Chapter 9: Kitchen Tools & Appliance List 123

Introduction

Welcome to the world of Figure Friendly Meals in Minutes. This will possibly be one of the more non-traditional cookbooks that you've read. This book was designed for you, the person on the go who wants to be able to quickly get delicious, Figure Friendly, family-style meals on the table while only investing mere minutes each day.

In the pages that follow, you won't find fancy recipes with exotic ingredients or complex cooking techniques. You won't even need to break out your measuring spoons. We measure by the shake around here. It's faster, and it still gets the job done.

What you will find in the pages that follow are realistic meal guidelines to help you create meals that taste great and help you get results, cooking strategy to cut down your time in the kitchen, delicious recipes, and resources that help you go beyond the recipes in this book to create your own.

Each recipe in the book includes detailed steps to ensure that your meal is prepped in minutes so that you are free to do other things with your time. Be sure to follow the steps as detailed because order matters. Ignoring the steps can significantly increase your meal preparation time.

If you find that it's taking longer than expected to prep the meals, try reading over the recipes before you start the meal prep. This way, you'll know what you're doing before you start. Also, it can be helpful to prepare the same meal more than once in a short time frame. Just like everything else in life, making meals in minutes gets easier with practice.

In the recipes, you'll encounter a few instructions that may be unfamiliar. To see video demonstrations of how to season using shakes or creating foil dividers, as mentioned in the recipes, be sure to visit concitathomas.com/bookextras.

My promise to you is that if you give these strategies a shot and consistently prepare the recipes in this book, you'll be able to get delicious, family-style, Figure Friendly Meals on your table in just minutes each day. You'll be done with the weekend meal prep forever. Even though the recipes are simple, they are delicious and healthy too. However, you can keep the health value of the meals to yourself if you have family members who are convinced that healthy meals aren't tasty. These recipes have been approved by my family, which includes my husband and two young children. I've even served some of the meals at parties and gotten rave reviews. My sincere hope is that your family will love them too.

Here's to a lifetime of reclaimed time and satisfied bellies in your home!

PART I

Guidelines & Strategies

A book of recipes can be helpful but understanding the guidelines and strategies behind the recipes is powerful. In this section of the book, you will learn why the meals are built the way they are and the strategies we use to make them quickly. This information will empower you to confidently tweak the recipes, as desired, to suit your preferences without compromising the Figure Friendly factor or efficiency of preparation.

Chapter 1

WHAT IS A FIGURE FRIENDLY MEAL?

Figure Friendly meals are meals that support overall health, performance and weight management. They aren't designed to optimize one over the other. If you've read more than one article or blog post about eating right, you've likely encountered conflicting information. Some may suggest that you reduce carbohydrates. Others may claim that eating only organic food is most important.

The truth is that to create positive outcomes in health, performance, and weight management, you must strike a balance and avoid extremes. There are meals that may positively improve your health outcomes that aren't ideal for weight loss. On the other hand, some meals that are promoted for weight loss, aren't healthy. Finally, meals that may be recommended to improve athletic performance would contribute to weight gain for the everyday woman who doesn't participate in a rigorous, high volume workout program or athletic pursuits. Figure Friendly eating is the sweet spot where you are eating to support those three main outcomes. Eating this way may not be ideal if you want to optimize one outcome without consideration for the others.

TYPES OF EATING STYLES

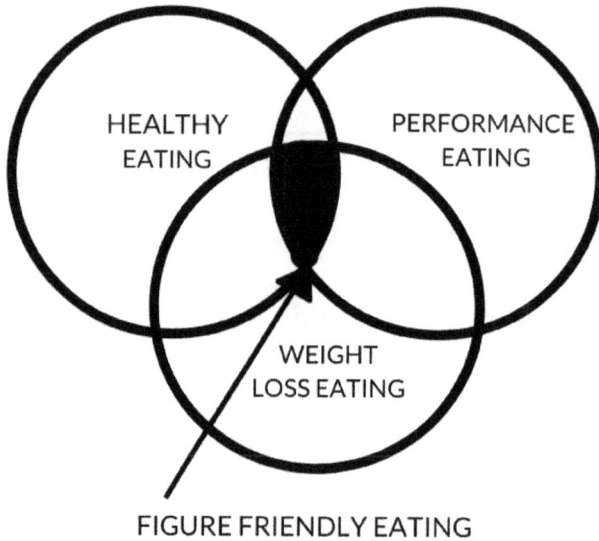

HEALTHY EATING

PERFORMANCE EATING

WEIGHT LOSS EATING

FIGURE FRIENDLY EATING

Figure Friendly Eating guidelines may contradict some of the beliefs you've held about eating right - and they should. If you've ever focused heavily on improved health, performance, or weight loss without a consideration for all three, then it's likely that some of the guidelines will surprise you. Let's get into what a day of Figure Friendly eating looks like.

Figure Friendly Eating Guidelines

- At least three servings of green vegetables
- At least 3L (96 ounces) of water
- Protein with each meal
- Fat or starch with each meal
- Minimal added sugar
- Minimal heavily processed food items

As you can tell from the guidelines, the focus of Figure Friendly Eating is an abundance of foods that are high in water, fiber, and protein with just enough of everything else to keep you satisfied. This style of eating is easily customized to suit individual preferences and needs. It's not low carb or low fat. It's balanced and adjustable.

Figure Friendly Eating is very different from other styles of eating which require that you eliminate or drastically reduce whole food groups. You'll also notice that, besides the specifications for water and green vegetables, there aren't any specific numbers- calories or grams- involved. That's because Figure Friendly Eating is not intended to place specific restrictions and calculations on you. There's no need to count and track food like a Food Accountant. You simply eat well balanced meals, pay attention to how your body feels and responds, and adjust from there. This is the exact approach that has helped my clients and I achieve lasting results.

Figure Friendly Meal Guidelines

Here are the components of a Figure Friendly Meal.

- Source of Protein (full portion)
- Source of Vegetables and/or Fruit
- Serving of Fat or Starch (not both)

Meals that produce sustainable results meet two needs. The meal helps you to feel full. It also helps you feel satisfied. Probably like you, I have eaten meals that filled me up but still left me desiring something else. That's what happens when you're full but not satisfied. On the other hand, I've experienced meals that made my taste buds dance and left me satisfied. However, the meals weren't filling. I was looking for something else to eat shortly after the meal. Figure Friendly Meals are designed to give you the best of both worlds- leaving you full and satisfied, but not stuffed.

To meet the two critical needs that a Figure Friendly Meal must meet, they have both fullness factors and satisfaction factors. The protein, vegetables, and fruit are the fullness factors in each meal. The combination of protein, fiber, and water from the vegetables and fruit fill your stomach. The satisfaction factors are starch and fat. Including a serving of either starch or fruit makes a filling meal more satisfactory. Choosing one or the other, rather than both, helps you feel full and satisfied without feeling stuffed. It's that simple.

Understanding which meal components serve which purpose allows you to customize your meals to meet your needs. If you're not feeling full after your meals, you simply add more vegetables or fruit first. Vegetables and fruit are filling with relatively few calories. If making that adjustment doesn't help you feel full, you simply increase the size of your protein portion. If you're not feeling satisfied after your meals, consider switching which satisfaction factor you include. For instance, you may find a fattier cut of meat more satisfying than a side of rice. This knowledge and methodical approach to adjusting your meals empowers you to create meals that leave you full and satisfied without compromising your results.

Chapter 2

THE MEALS IN MINUTES STRATEGY

How can I make dinner quickly? More importantly, how can I make a quick dinner that the entire family will eat? That is the dilemma. Before we can get into how to make dinner quickly, we must understand why making dinner takes so long. When we know why our current approach doesn't yield the results we want, we can simply do the opposite to get the results we want.

Why does dinner take so long in the first place?

There are a few major factors that contribute to a lengthy dinner prep. They are common traps that most of us have fallen into at some point in time. Recognizing and avoiding those traps is the key to making meals in minutes.

Our recipes are too complicated.

If you want to make your meals quickly, embrace simplicity. Recipes that require a long list of ingredients and multi-step cooking methods increase your time in the kitchen. Save complicated recipes for the weekend, holidays, or other times when you have extra time to spare.

The Solution: Choose recipes with a short ingredients list and minimal steps.

Each item in the meal should be fully prepared in just a few steps. We can boil steam, sauté, fry, or bake. However, any one item won't need multiple different methods. For example, meatballs and roasted chicken are excellent choices for quick meals because they require minimal preparation before being placed in the oven. For meatballs, the meat only needs to be seasoned and formed. For roasted chicken, the chicken only needs to be washed and seasoned. Preparation is straightforward and quick so that you can create your meal in minutes.

We also want to eventually eliminate the need to measure ingredients. Have you ever watched an experienced cook prepare a meal? If you have, you've probably noticed that they don't measure ingredients. One example of a great cook that stood out to me from an early age was my Granny Lou. Her food was amazing, but the thing that intrigued me the most was watching her cook. She would taste something and immediately know if it "needed a little something". She also seemed to magically know which little something it needed - without measuring spoons. Even if you don't want to be a great cook like my granny, getting to the point where you don't need to precisely measure ingredients is both freeing and time saving.

While we want to start with recipes to become familiar with different flavor combinations and to learn which herbs and spices taste good together, we don't want to need a recipe forever. That may sound ambitious, but it's possible. This book will help.

Our recipes aren't familiar.

It's both a blessing and a curse to live in a time where we have so much information available to us at the push of a button. Just a few minutes spent searching Pinterest can yield several meal ideas that we now feel inspired to cook-right away. This inspiration toward endless variety costs us our time. It takes longer to cook a meal for the first time. We spend extra time making sure that we are taking the proper steps and using the correct amount of each ingredient. When we want to prepare meals in minutes, an unfamiliar recipe is an obstacle to be avoided.

The Solution: Build a roster of familiar recipes and add to that roster slowly and intentionally.

This recommendation probably seems strange. After all, this is a cookbook filled with fifty recipes that are likely new to you. However, you can still follow this advice. When it comes to the recipes in this book, start with the ones that are like things you've cooked in the past. That will give you the best chance or preparing them quickly- even the first time. When you've mastered a group of four to five recipes, keep things fresh by rotating in one new recipe each week. Instead of adding a new recipe that is completely different than any of your usual ones, pick one that is only slightly different as your new addition to the rotation.

In this book, you'll find several meals that have completely different flavors but only differ slightly in terms of preparation and ingredients. Sometimes the protein, starch, and vegetable are the same, but the seasonings make the difference. In other cases, the starch, vegetable, or seasonings are all different, but the preparation methods are the same. Those commonalities cultivate familiarity and save time.

One example of a meal pair that you can use to employ this strategy is the Asian and Mediterranean Meatball pair in this book. The meatball preparation is the same, but the spices are different. Even though the vegetables are different, the preparation technique is the same. The starches are different as well. However, the similarities are strong enough that mastery in preparation of one of the meals seamlessly transitions to the other. Making these subtle changes is how you'll save time while keeping an interesting weekly menu.

We spend a lot of time on ingredient prep.

Imagine that you've been working diligently in the kitchen for the last fifteen minutes and your big accomplishment is that the vegetables and herbs are prepared for use. Would you be happy about that on a busy weeknight? Probably not. That's what happens to so many of us when we decide to commit to making home cooked meals.

I often joke that I save the slicing and dicing for the holidays. However, that joke is almost entirely true. As a matter of fact, there was one holiday that I didn't slice a thing. I was visiting at my brother's house for Thanksgiving a few years ago. I was prepared to stay awake into the wee hours of the morning to help him cook because we hadn't started a single dish by nine o'clock the night before. I imagined that we would slice and dice herbs and vegetables for hours as I had done with my mom when I was younger. Imagine my surprise when he started pulling containers of diced onions, celery, and herbs out of the refrigerator. I was equally appalled and relieved, and I think he could see it on my face. He just smirked at me and kept preparing the meal.

Until that year, I had associated buying diced vegetables with cutting corners. I had convinced myself that the food wouldn't taste the same if you bought those things. Well, to my shock, the vegetables and herbs were extremely fresh, and the food tasted just as good as it always had in previous years. The only difference was that we were well rested when dinnertime arrived because we hadn't spent the entire night slicing and dicing. That experience made me a believer when it comes to buying partially prepared ingredients. I'll admit that I still slice and dice a lot of my own ingredients during the holiday season. I think it's just nostalgic. However, I don't do that for my regular weekday meals anymore. If you want to make meals in minutes, you won't either.

The Solution: Buy food items that are partially prepared.

15

These days we have partially prepared, fresh food items available in almost every grocery store. We can buy diced onions, minced garlic, and flash frozen broccoli crowns. These items end up tasting just as good as fresh items that require full preparation. This same approach carries over to our meat. We don't have to buy a whole chicken only to have to cut it, clean it, and remove the fat ourselves. We can buy chicken pieces or boneless skinless chicken breasts. When we do, we only need to wash it and season it before putting it in the oven. This is how we shave minutes off our cooking process and create delicious meals with just a little time in the kitchen each day.

Partially prepared food can be leveraged as much or as little as we like. There are many options beyond purchasing skinless meat and chopped vegetables. We can also purchase seasoned meat and precooked rice blends. When we purchase those items, meal preparation can be as simple as placing the meat in the oven and the starch in the microwave. How far you go with partially prepared items is up to you. Honor your personal preferences and have fun with this.

If you remember nothing else, remember this. If you make one item that requires a little more preparation, make sure that the rest of the items are simple. For example, in the Mediterranean Meatballs meal in this book, forming the meatballs is an extra step when you compare that meal to meals with roasted meat pieces. To offset the extra time spent forming the meatballs, we pair that dish with rice and green beans. Both of those items require zero prep before cooking. I purposely resisted the urge to pair the meatballs with roasted potatoes. While that combination is delicious, it's time consuming. The potatoes must be sliced before being placed in the oven. Pairing those items together in one meal would increase the active cooking time required in the meal. So, remember, no more than one moderately complicated item in a meal.

We aren't using the right tools for the job or we're not using any tools at all.

Have you ever tried to cut a potato with a dull knife? I have. I can tell you that it takes much longer than doing it with a sharp knife, and you run a higher risk of cutting yourself. The right tools make all the difference when it comes to preparing meals efficiently. Sometimes the right tool isn't so obvious. I can remember the first time that I peeled a cucumber with a potato peeler. I was amazed that it could be done so quickly.

In this book, if it matters, I mention which tools you should use to do a job. Pay attention to those recommendations because they are there to help you save time. You'll notice that I use a few appliances often in the recipes that follow. Use the same appliances when you can. Resist the urge to just cook the items on the stove top instead. When we insist on standing over the stove like our grandmothers did, it's hard to create meals in minutes. Maybe, like I did with the pre-cut vegetables, you associate kitchen appliances with cutting corners and creating less than delicious dishes. With the advances in technology, that's simply not the case anymore.

The Solution: Leverage kitchen tools to reduce active cooking time.

The days of standing over the stove to cook like our grandmothers did are over. Unless it's a holiday, a special occasion, or you find it extremely relaxing to do, it's completely unnecessary. My guess is that if you found cooking extremely relaxing, you wouldn't have even purchased this book. Leverage the kitchen tools that you already have. Also, assess your needs to identify the kitchen tools that may be worth purchasing in in the future to make your cooking process a lot quicker each day. In another chapter, I provide a detailed outline of which tools I use to do which jobs in the kitchen. However, you don't have to buy everything I mention.

If you have an oven and a few baking tools, you have enough to get off to a great start. All the kitchen tools can be leveraged to significantly reduce your cooking time without sacrificing flavor or compromising the nutrition value of your food.

We aren't completing steps in an order that leverages downtime in the cooking process.

Instead of strategically cooking things in an order that reduces prep time, we prepare items randomly or in order to have everything finish at the same time. When your goal is to cook meal in minutes, cooking order is critically important. The goal is to never be standing around waiting. You either want to be cooking or moving on to something else while your kitchen tools finish cooking what you've prepared.

The Solution: Follow a cooking order that allows you to make use of downtime in the process.

The specific order you follow will vary from meal to meal. The exact order to follow is specified for each recipe in this book. However, a general rule of thumb is to start any meal that will require baking or boiling by turning on the water and preheating the oven first. While the oven and water are heating, you can slice any vegetables that aren't pre-sliced and wash and season the meat. By the time you finish these tasks, the water and oven will be ready for use. This is a simple strategy that saves a tremendous amount of time.

We're trying too hard to be creative in pursuit of variety.

Do you have a pantry full of half used items? Do you routinely have to clear your refrigerator of spoiled food that never made it to the stove? If so, this could be a sign that you're trying too hard in your pursuit of variety. Most of us don't want to eat the same exact meal every single night. However, when our pursuit of variety leads us to make meals that we never make again and buy ingredients that can't be used in multiple meals, we'll probably have a lot of wasted time to match those wasted ingredients.

The Solution: Create meals that use the same proteins, starches, and vegetables, but different spices and herbs.

You'll notice that the same handful of meats, vegetables, and starches appear in this book again and again. That's not due to a lack of creativity on my part. I use the same items again and again to keep things simple and to show you just how much variety you can create with a few simple variations in spice and preparation methods.

We aren't doing things in an organized, methodical fashion.

Have you ever ended up ordering take out because everything was frozen when you were ready to cook? Have you ever burned your rice while you searched for the pan to cook the chicken? These scenarios are signs of a disorganized cooking process. This lack of organization and lack of process makes meal prep less efficient.

The Solution: Leverage the Morning Thaw and an equipped meal prep station.

One of the simplest ways to decrease your cooking time is to get everything ready before you start. By before you start, I mean when you wake up in the morning. In the morning, one of the first things I do when I emerge from my bedroom is to take the meat for dinner out of the freezer. I've done that so consistently now that it is as automatic as brushing my teeth. It happens as my coffee is brewing, right after I put the day's load of laundry into the washing machine. Your morning routine may be a little different from mine. However, the easiest way to remember to practice The Morning Thaw is to link taking the meat out of the freezer to something that you do every morning- preferably something that you do in the kitchen.

When it's time to cook, do it like the pros. You've probably watched at least one cooking show at some point in your life. Have you ever noticed that they never have to go looking for a pot, pan, spoon, or spice? If you thought that approach was only for TV, you may want to reconsider that position. Although it may seem counterintuitive to have so many things on the counter at once, equipping your meal prep station before you start cooking saves loads of time. You're able to move from one task to another without losing time looking for the things that you need. What's even better is that you'll realize if you don't have something you need before you have pots on the stove and food in the oven. You'll be able to either make a quick switch or send someone to the store before you start cooking.

We don't have a plan.

It's almost as if dinnertime takes us by surprise. We glance at the clock and break out into a frenzy trying to figure out what we'll cook that night. All of that scurrying and scrambling is wasted time. Maybe you don't waste time when you fail to plan. Maybe, like I used to, you just dial one of your many go to restaurants to order takeout. To be honest, ordering takeout isn't the worst thing that you can do. As a matter of fact, when you know how to place a Figure Friendly order, takeout can save you when you're in a pinch. However, when you order dinner most nights of the week for months on end, you eventually want home cooked food. Well, at least that's what happened in my case. If you're at that place where you want home cooked food more often than you want takeout, you need a plan to help you save time.

For a while, I resisted the planning process because I knew that I could get Figure Friendly food anywhere. You learned the Figure Friendly Meal guidelines in the last chapter. I'm sure if you think about it, you can think of a way to order a meal that falls into those guidelines, too. After years of participating in bodybuilding competitions and meal prepping for hours each Sunday even after I stopped competing, I didn't want to plan my food. I enjoyed the variety and spontaneity of ordering my food or just cooking whatever I had a taste for on any given night. However, when my evening calendar began filling up with more after school activities, I knew it was time to try a different way. I still didn't want to do a weekly meal prep. However, I needed to embrace a Weekly Menu Plan.

The Solution: Create a *Weekly Menu Plan.*

We can feel calm and prepared at dinner time by creating a Weekly Menu Plan. Before talking about the plan, let's address the obvious. If you wanted to spend time planning meals for an entire week, you wouldn't have purchased this book. Right? I get it. The traditional way that we've been taught to menu plan is time consuming. However, there is a more efficient way. Want to hear about it? Here it goes. (I hope you caught that reference. If not, just know that you were supposed to laugh right there.)

How do I decided what to cook for an entire week?
The menu planning process starts with accessing what you already have in your house and which types of flavors you want to enjoy that week. Start by deciding which protein sources you want to have that week. Next, decide which types of cuisine you want. Nailing down those two components makes the rest of the process go quickly. We've already discussed the importance of having only one meal component that takes more than two steps of preparation before it can be placed in the oven or other kitchen appliance to cook. So, if your protein choice is that item, you'll know that your starch and vegetable selections must be simple. Let's look at a couple of examples. In our Asian Meatballs meal, the meatball must be seasoned and formed. Forming the meatballs takes a little bit of extra

time. So, we paired them with pot stickers and broccoli. Both of those go straight from the package to the stove with no additional prep. In our Rosemary Chicken meal, the chicken is only washed and seasoned before being placed in the oven. That takes less than five minutes, so we have a little extra time to spare for the starch and vegetable prep. We pair the chicken with roasted potatoes. They must be washed, sliced, and seasoned before being placed in the oven. However, we have the time because the chicken required so little prep. See how this works?

The meals in this book were created with efficiency in mind. So, you won't have to think about this if all your meals for the week are from this book. However, there's one more step that you can take in creating your Weekly Menu Plan to best compliment your life.

Plan the simplest meals for the busiest days. You may want to pick a meal that consists of all low prep items or a one pot meal on nights that you know you have even less time. Meals like Chicken Tortilla Soup and One Pot Chicken are perfect options for busy nights.

Figure Friendly Meals in Minutes Cooking Strategy

1. Make meals from simple recipes with minimal ingredients and steps.
2. Master a small set of recipes first then add no more than one new recipe each week.
3. Buy food items that are partially prepped.
4. Acquire a few key kitchen tools to reduce active cooking time.
5. Prep meal components in an order that leverages the downtime in the cooking process.
6. To create a meal, pick a protein, starch, and vegetable. Create variety with spices and herbs.
7. Set yourself up for efficiency with the Morning Thaw strategy and an equipped meal prep station.
8. Create a Weekly Menu Plan.

PART II

The Recipes

This section provides you with 50 recipes to take the guesswork out of applying the Figure Friendly Meal guidelines and Meals in Minutes Cooking Strategy. In this section, you will find diverse meals with complete cooking instructions to help you prepare fresh meals in just minutes each day.

Chapter 3

CHICKEN

- Rosemary Chicken & Roasted Potatoes with Green Beans
- Jerk Chicken & Plantains with Shredded Cabbage
- Oven Fajitas & Southwest Salad
- BBQ Chicken & Yams with Green Beans
- Thai Curry Chicken & Rice
- Puerto Rican Chicken & Rice with Tomato Cucumber Salad
- Italian Chicken & Potatoes with Asparagus
- Asian Chicken & Rice with Broccoli
- Chicken Stew
- Mediterranean Chicken & Roasted Cauliflower with Caesar Salad
- Fried Chicken & Yams with Green Beans
- Chicken Parmesan & Roasted Potatoes with Broccolini
- Chicken Tortilla Soup

Rosemary Chicken & Roasted Potatoes with Green Beans

Active Cooking: 7 min | Total Cooking: 52 min |Serves 4

Appliances: Oven

Ingredients:

- 1 lb. chicken, cut in pieces
- 1 lemon
- 13 shakes salt, divided
- 10 shakes garlic powder
- 13 shakes lemon pepper, divided
- 5 sprigs rosemary
- 1 lb. whole green beans, frozen
- 6 small potatoes, sliced

Directions:

1. Preheat the oven to 350F. Place a medium pot half full of water over high heat to bring to a boil.
2. In a large bowl, wash the chicken with water and the juice of a lemon. Then, rinse and drain. Season the chicken with 5 shakes each of salt, garlic powder, and lemon pepper on each side. Place the chicken on a foil lined baking sheet and top with rosemary sprigs.
3. Meanwhile, the water has come to a boil. Pour the green beans into the pot and continue to cook on high heat.
4. Next, rinse and peel the potatoes. Slice the potatoes into ½-inch thick slices and place them on a foil lined baking sheet coated with cooking spray. Season

the potatoes with 3 shakes each of salt and lemon pepper and toss. Spray the exposed side of the potatoes with cooking spray.

5. Place the chicken and potatoes in the oven and set a timer for 25 minutes.
6. Remove the pot from the stove. Drain the green beans and cover to keep warm.

Your active cooking is done!
Let your appliances do the rest!

When the timer alarms, remove the potatoes from the oven. Cover with foil to keep warm. Set another timer for 20 minutes. After 20 minutes, remove the chicken from the oven.

---------- *Figure Friendly Meal Notes* ----------

This Figure Friendly Meal includes starch as the satisfaction factor. If you're more satisfied by fat, eliminate the potatoes and drizzle olive oil on your green beans.

Jerk Chicken & Plantains
with Shredded Cabbage

Active Cooking: 7 min | Total Cooking: 47 min | Serves 4

Appliances: Oven

Ingredients:

- 1 lb. chicken, cut in pieces
- 1 lime
- 2 spoonsful jerk seasoning, paste
- 10 shakes season salt
- 10 shakes garlic powder
- 2 large plantains, ripe
- 1 spoonful coconut oil
- 2 bags (10 oz) shredded cabbage

Directions:

1. Preheat the oven to 350F.
2. In a large bowl, wash the chicken with water and the juice of a lime. Then, rinse and drain. Season the chicken with 5 shakes each of season salt and garlic powder on both sides. Then, stir in the jerk seasoning with a large spoon. Continue stirring until it is evenly distributed. Place the chicken on a foil lined baking sheet.
3. Next, cut off the tip from both sides of the plantain. Run a knife lengthwise through the skin without cutting through the flesh. Then, remove the skin from side to side- instead of lengthwise. Cut the plantains into ½ -inch thick slices before placing them on a foil lined baking sheet coated with cooking spray. Spray the exposed side of the plantains with cooking spray.
4. Place the plantains and chicken in the oven and set a timer for 15 minutes.
5. Melt one spoonful of coconut oil in a pan over high heat. When warm, add the shredded cabbage and sauté until cabbage starts to wilt, 3 minutes. Then,

add just enough water to cover the bottom of the pan. Reduce to low heat. Cover the pan and simmer for 5 minutes before removing from heat.

Your active cooking is done! Let your appliances do the rest!

When the timer alarms, flip the plantains to the other side, and set another timer for 25 minutes. When the timer alarms again, remove the chicken and plantains from the oven. Plantains will be browned and easily penetrated with a fork.

---------- *Figure Friendly Meal Notes* ----------

This Figure Friendly Meal includes starch as the satisfaction factor. If you're more satisfied by fat, eliminate the plantains and be more liberal with the coconut oil in the cabbage, or enjoy a few avocado slices with the meal instead.

Oven Fajitas & Southwest Salad

Active Cooking: 4 min | Total Cooking: 44 min | Serves 4

Appliances Used: Oven

Ingredients:

- 1 lb. chicken breast, boneless skinless
- 1 lime

- 10 shakes salt
- 10 shakes garlic powder
- 14 shakes cumin
- 3 green bell peppers, sliced
- 1 onion, sliced
- 1 Southwest Salad Kit
- 8 medium (8-inch) tortillas

Directions:

1. Preheat the oven to 350F.
2. In a large bowl, wash the chicken with water and the juice of a lime. Then, rinse and drain. Season the chicken with 5 shakes each of salt and garlic powder and 7 shakes of cumin on each side. Place the chicken on a foil lined baking sheet. Top the chicken with bell pepper and onion slices. Then, place the chicken in the oven and set a timer for 40 minutes.
3. Open the salad kit and mix according to the instructions on the package.

Your active cooking is done!
Let your appliances do the rest!

Remove the chicken from the oven after 40 minutes. Slice the chicken into large pieces and serve with tortillas.

---------- *Figure Friendly Meal Notes* ----------

While this meal is generally Figure Friendly, you'll have to choose your meal components wisely to avoid consuming full portions of both satisfaction factors, starch and fat, in the same meal. If you're most satisfied by starch, enjoy both tortillas but use the dressing in the salad kit sparingly to reduce the amount of fat in the meal. However, if you're most satisfied by fat, prepare the salad kit with all the dressing provided, use half of the tortilla chips in the kit, and skip the tortillas. Also, feel free to use salsa liberally. If you choose to add cheese or sour cream (sources of fat), add no more than 2 spoonsful total or eliminate the tortillas and enjoy more of these condiments.

BBQ Chicken & Yams with Green Beans

Active Cooking: 6 min | Total Cooking: 40 min | Serves 4

Appliances: Oven

Ingredients:

- 2 large yams
- 1 lb. whole green beans, frozen
- 1 whole chicken, cut in pieces
- 1 lemon
- 10 shakes season salt
- 14 shakes garlic powder
- 4 shakes black pepper
- BBQ sauce

Directions:

1. Preheat the oven to 350F. Fill a medium pot half full of water over high heat to bring to a boil.

2. While rinsing with water, rub yams vigorously to remove dirt. Place yams on a foil lined baking sheet and use a fork to poke holes in the yams on all sides.
3. Meanwhile, the water has come to a boil. Pour the green beans into the boiling water and continue to cook on high heat.
4. In a large bowl, wash the chicken with water and the juice of a lemon. Then, rinse and drain. Season the chicken with the 5 shakes of season salt, 7 shakes of garlic powder, and 2 shakes of black pepper on each side. Then, place the chicken in a baking dish and pour ½ bottle of the BBQ sauce on the chicken.
5. Cover the dish with foil. Then, place the chicken and yams in the oven and set a timer for 40 minutes.
6. Meanwhile, the green beans have cooked. Drain and cover to keep warm.

Your active cooking is done!
Let your appliances do the rest!

When the timer alarms, remove the chicken and yams from the oven. The yams should have a brown syrup seeping out of them. If not, leave them in the oven until this happens.

---------- *Figure Friendly Meal Notes* ----------

This Figure Friendly Meal includes starch as the satisfaction factor. If you're more satisfied by fat, skip the yam and be more liberal with the butter in the green beans.

Thai Curry Chicken & Rice

Active Cooking: 4 min | Total Cooking: 8 hrs 4 min | Serves 4

Appliances: Pressure Cooker, Crockpot

Ingredients:

- 1 cup rice
- 2 cups water
- 1 lb. chicken tenderloins
- 1 lb. green beans, frozen
- 10 shakes salt
- 10 shakes garlic powder
- 14 shakes umami seasoning
- 1 bottle yellow Thai curry sauce

Directions:

1. Place the rice and water in the pressure cooker. Set it for 4 minutes on the manual setting.
2. In a large bowl, wash the chicken with water. Then, rinse and drain. Slice the chicken strips horizontally into ½-inch thick slices.
3. Place all the ingredients in the Crockpot. Then, stir to combine ingredients. Cook in the crock pot on low for 6-8 hours or on high for 3-4 hours.

Your active cooking is done!
Let your appliances do the rest!

When you're ready to eat, remove the meal from the Crockpot.

---------- *Figure Friendly Meal Notes* ----------

This Figure Friendly Meal includes starch as the satisfaction factor. If you're more satisfied by fat, skip the rice. Eat the chicken like stew and have dark chocolate for dessert.

Puerto Rican Chicken & Rice
with Tomato Cucumber Salad

Active Cooking: 5 min | Total Cooking: 45 min | Serves 4

Appliances Used: Oven, Pressure Cooker

Ingredients:

- 1 cup rice
- 2 cups water
- 1 whole chicken, cut in pieces
- 1 lime, whole
- 10 shakes salt
- 10 shakes garlic powder
- 14 shakes oregano
- 14 shakes cumin
- 8 shakes paprika
- 3 cucumbers
- 2 Roma tomatoes

Directions:

1. Preheat the oven to 350F. Pour the rice and water into the pressure cooker. Set for 4 minutes on the manual setting.
2. In a large bowl, wash the chicken in water and the juice of a lime. Then, rinse and drain. Season the chicken with 5 shakes each of salt and garlic powder, 7 shakes each of oregano and cumin, and 4 shakes of paprika on each side.
3. Place the chicken on a foil lined baking sheet and place in the oven. Set a timer for 40 minutes.
4. Rinse the cucumber and tomato with water. Peel the cucumbers with a potato peeler. Run a knife down the length of each cucumber to cut in half. Next, cut the cucumbers in ½-inch slices. Run a knife down the length of each tomato to cut in half. Next, cut the tomatoes into ½-inch thick slices. Combine the cucumber and tomato slices in a bowl and toss.

Your active cooking is done!
Let your appliances do the rest!

When the timer alarms, remove the chicken from the oven. Drizzle your favorite dressing on top of the salad.

---------- *Figure Friendly Meal Notes* ----------

This Figure Friendly Meal includes starch as the satisfaction factor. If you're more satisfied by fat, skip the rice and add avocado slices or a higher fat dressing to the salad.

Italian Chicken & Potatoes with Asparagus

Active Cooking: 5 min | Total Cooking: 45 min | Serves 4

Appliances: Oven

Ingredients:

- 8 potatoes, small golden
- 13 shakes salt, divided
- 17 shakes oregano, divided
- 1 bunch asparagus
- 1 lb. chicken breasts
- 10 shakes garlic powder

Directions:

1. Preheat the oven to 350F.
2. Rinse the potatoes with water while rubbing them vigorously to remove dirt. Next, cut them into ½ -inch thick slices. Place the potatoes on a foil lined baking sheet that is coated with cooking spray and season with 3 shakes each of salt and oregano. Toss then spray the exposed side with cooking spray.
3. Rinse the asparagus spears and place them on the same foil lined baking sheet as the potatoes. Use a foil divider to separate the two items.
4. In a large bowl, wash the chicken with water. Then, rinse and drain. Season the chicken with 5 shakes each of salt and garlic powder and 7 shakes of oregano on each side. Place the chicken on a foil lined baking sheet.
5. Place all the food in the oven and set a timer for 10 minutes.

Your active cooking is done!
Let your appliances do the rest!

When the timer alarms, remove the asparagus from the oven. Cover with foil to keep warm and set another timer for 30 minutes. When the final timer alarms, remove the chicken and potatoes form the oven.

---------- *Figure Friendly Meal Notes* ----------

This Figure Friendly Meal includes starch as the satisfaction factor. If you're more satisfied by fat, skip the potatoes and drizzle olive oil on your asparagus.

Asian Chicken & Rice with Broccoli

Active Cooking: 5 min | Total Cooking: 45 min | Serves 4

Appliances: Oven, Pressure Cooker

Ingredients:

- 1 cup rice
- 2 cups water
- 1 whole chicken, cut in pieces
- 1 lemon, whole
- 10 shakes salt
- 10 shakes garlic
- 10 umami seasoning
- soyaki sauce

- 1 lb. broccoli, frozen

Directions:

1. Preheat the oven to 350F. Place medium pot half full of water on the stove over high heat to bring to a boil. Place the rice and water into the pressure cooker. Set for 4 minutes on manual setting.
2. In a large bowl, wash the chicken with water. Then, rinse and drain. Season chicken with 5 shakes each of salt, garlic powder, and umami. Place the chicken in a baking dish and cover with soyaki sauce.
3. Place the chicken in the oven and set a timer for 40 minutes.
4. Meanwhile, the water has come to a boil. Pour the broccoli in the pot and continue to cook over high heat.

Your active cooking is done!
Let your appliances do the rest!

After 5 minutes, drain the broccoli and cover to keep warm. When the timer alarms, remove the chicken from the oven.

---------- *Figure Friendly Meal Notes* ----------

This is a Figure Friendly Meal which includes starch as the satisfaction factor. If you're most satisfied with fat, skip the rice and add butter to your broccoli instead.

_____

Chicken Stew

Active Cooking: 5 min | Total Cooking: 8 hrs 5 min | Serves 4

Appliances: Crockpot

Ingredients:

- 8 potatoes, small golden
- 1 lb. chicken tenderloins
- 1 lb. green beans, frozen
- ½ package (16 oz) baby carrots
- 2 spoonsful salt
- 3 spoonsful garlic powder
- 2 spoonsful onion powder
- 2 spoonsful black pepper
- 2 cups chicken broth

Directions:

1. While rinsing them with water, rub the potatoes vigorously to remove dirt. Cut them into ½-inch slices.
2. In a large bowl, wash the chicken with water. Then, rinse and drain. Slice the chicken strips horizontally into ½-inch slices.
3. Place all the ingredients in the Crockpot. Then, stir to mix the ingredients well. Cook in the crock pot on low for 6-8 hours or on high for 2-3 hours

Your active cooking is done!
Let your appliances do the rest!

When you're ready to eat, remove the meal from the Crockpot.

---------- *Figure Friendly Meal Notes* ----------

This Figure Friendly Meal contains starch as the satisfaction factor. If you're more satisfied by fat, skip the potatoes, and have some dark chocolate for dessert.

Mediterranean Chicken & Roasted Cauliflower with Caesar Salad

Active Cooking: 5 min | Total Cooking: 45 min | Serves 4

Appliances: Oven

Ingredients:

- 2 bags (10 oz) cauliflower florets
- 15 shakes salt, divided
- 15 shakes garlic powder, divided
- olive oil
- 1 lb. chicken, cut in pieces
- 1 lemon
- 14 shakes lemon pepper
- 10 shakes cumin
- 1 Caesar Salad Kit

Directions:

1. Preheat the oven to 350F.
2. Rinse the cauliflower florets. Place them on a foil lined baking sheet and season with 5 shakes each of garlic powder and salt. Drizzle olive oil on the cauliflower and toss.
3. In a large bowl, wash the chicken with water and the juice of a lemon. Then, rinse and drain. Season the chicken with 5 shakes each of salt, garlic powder, and cumin as well as 7 shakes of lemon pepper on each side. Next, place the chicken on a foil lined baking sheet.
4. Place the chicken and cauliflower in the oven. Set a timer for 30 minutes.
5. Open the Caesar Salad Kit and prepare according to the instructions on the package.

Your active cooking is done!
Let your appliances do the rest!

When the timer alarms, remove the cauliflower from the oven. Set another timer for 10 minutes. When the timer alarms, remove the chicken from the oven.

---------- *Figure Friendly Meal Notes* ----------

This Figure Friendly meal includes fat as the satisfaction factor. If you're more satisfied by starch, include a serving of rice. Then, use cooking spray on the cauliflower instead of olive oil and approximately half of the dressing that comes with the salad kit in order to reduce the fat content of the meal.

Fried Chicken & Yams with Green Beans

Active Cooking: 10 min | Total Cooking: 45 min | Serves 4

Appliances Used: Oven, Air Fryer

Ingredients:

- 4 medium yams
- 1 lb. whole green beans, frozen
- 4 chicken quarters
- 10 shakes season salt
- 10 shakes garlic powder
- 6 shakes black pepper
- 1 egg
- 1 cup milk
- ½ package (9 oz) chicken fry mix

Directions:

1. Preheat oven to 350F. Preheat air fryer to 400F. Place medium pot half full of water on the stove over high heat to bring to a boil.
2. Rinse the yams with water while rubbing vigorously to remove dirt. Place the yams on a foil lined baking sheet. Next, use a fork to poke holes in them in several places. Place the yams into the oven and set a timer for 35 minutes.
3. Meanwhile, the water has come to a boil. Add the green beans to the pot and continue to cook on high heat.
4. In a large bowl, wash chicken in water. Then, rinse and drain. Season chicken with 5 shakes each of season salt, and garlic powder as well as 3 shakes of

black pepper per side. In a shallow bowl, crack and beat an egg. Then, add milk and mix to combine ingredients. Place the chicken fry mix on a plate and spread it out evenly.

5. Dip each piece of chicken, one at a time, in the egg and milk mixture then immediately press it into the chicken fry mix to coat the chicken. Next, press the other side of the chicken into the chicken fry mix to coat. Finally, place coated chicken on a plate.

6. By now, the green beans are bright green and soft. Remove the green beans from the stove. Drain and cover to keep warm.

7. When all the chicken is coated, spray the inside of the air fryer with cooking spray and then place the chicken in the fryer. Spray cooking spray on the exposed side of the chicken. Then, close the fryer and set for 20 minutes.

Your active cooking is done!
Let your appliances do the rest!

When the chicken is done, remove from the fryer. When the timer alarms, remove yams from the oven. You should see brown syrup running out of the yams. This is your sign that they are not only done but also sweet.

---------- *Figure Friendly Meal Notes* ----------

This Figure Friendly meal includes starch as the satisfaction factor. If you're more satisfied by fat, skip the yams, and add butter or olive oil to your green beans instead.

Chicken Parmesan & Roasted Potatoes with Broccolini

Active Cooking: 6 min | Total Cooking: 31 min | Serves 4

Appliances: Oven

Ingredients:

- 1 bunch broccolini
- 4 shakes lemon pepper
- 8 small potatoes, golden
- 15 shakes oregano, divided
- 15 shakes garlic powder, divided
- 15 shakes season salt, divided
- 4 medium chicken breasts, skinless boneless
- 6 shakes black pepper
- ½ bottle (16 oz) basil marinara sauce
- parmesan cheese, to taste

Directions:

1. Preheat the oven to 375F.
2. Rinse broccolini with water. Season it with 4 shakes of lemon pepper and place it on a foil lined baking sheet coated with cooking spray. Spray the exposed side of the broccolini with cooking spray.
3. While rinsing the potatoes with water, rub vigorously to remove dirt. Cut the potatoes into ½-inch slices. Season with 5 shakes each of oregano, garlic powder, and season salt. Then, place them on the same foil lined baking sheet as the broccolini. Use a foil divider to keep them separate.

4. Season chicken with 5 shakes each of season salt, garlic powder, and oregano as well as 3 shakes of black pepper on each side. Place chicken in a baking dish and cover with marinara sauce.
5. Place the chicken, potatoes, and broccolini in the oven, and set a timer for 15 minutes.

**Your active cooking is done!
Let your appliances do the rest!**

When the timer alarms, remove the broccolini and potatoes from the oven. Cover with foil to keep warm and set another timer for 7 minutes. When the timer alarms, remove the chicken from oven and sprinkle parmesan cheese on top. Let stand until cheese melts, 3 minutes.

---------- *Figure Friendly Meal Notes* ----------

This Figure Friendly Meal includes starch as the satisfaction factor. If you're more satisfied by fat, skip the potatoes and either drizzle olive oil on your broccolini or top your chicken with additional cheese.

Chicken Tortilla Soup

Active Cooking: 5 min | Total Cooking: 8 hrs 5 min | Serves 4

Appliances: Crockpot

Ingredients:

- 4 chicken breasts, boneless skinless (1 lb.)
- ½ package (16 oz) carrots, frozen
- 1 onion, chopped
- 1 package sweet corn, frozen
- 1 can Rotel, mild
- 1 can (14.5 oz) chicken broth
- 1 cup water
- 2 sprigs cilantro
- 2 spoonsful chili powder
- 2 spoonsful sea salt
- 2 spoonsful cumin
- tortilla chips, crushed

Directions:

1. In a large bowl, wash the chicken with water. Then, rinse and drain.
2. Place all the ingredients into a Crockpot. Stir to mix ingredients well. Cook on low for 8 hours or on high for 4 hours.

Your active cooking is done!
Let your appliances do the rest!

When the cooking time is complete, use two forks to shred the chicken that is in the slow cooker. Then, stir to evenly distribute the chicken again. Serve the soup in a bowl topped with crushed tortilla chips.

---------- *Figure Friendly Meal Notes* ----------

This Figure Friendly Meal doesn't include a significant source of either satisfaction factor, starch or fat. If you're more satisfied by starch, top each bowl of soup with approximately half-cup of tortilla chips (about 20 chips). If you're more satisfied by fat, top the soup with slices of avocado or cheese.

Chapter 4

GROUND MEAT

- Asian Meatballs & Pot Stickers with Broccoli
- Korean Beef Bowl
- Lettuce Wraps
- Meatloaf & Roasted Potatoes with Asparagus
- Sweet Basil Spaghetti & Simple Salad
- Italian Sausage & Peppers with Rice
- Mediterranean Meatballs & Rice with Green Beans
- Nachos
- Tacos & Cabbage Salad
- Bunless Burger & Fries with Broccoli Slaw
- Concita's Kicking Chili
- Sweet Potato Chili Boats & Simple Salad

Asian Meatballs & Pot Stickers with Broccoli

Active Cooking: 5 min | Total Cooking: 25 min | Serves 4

Appliances: Oven

Ingredients:

- 1 lb. lean ground meat (turkey, chicken, or beef)
- 10 shakes garlic powder
- 10 shakes umami seasoning
- 6 shakes season salt
- sweet chili sauce
- 1 lb. broccoli florets, frozen
- 1 package (16 oz) pot stickers

Directions:

1. Preheat the oven to 350F. Fill a medium pot half full of water and place over high heat to bring to a boil.
2. Season the ground meat with 5 shakes each of garlic powder and umami seasoning as well as 3 shakes of season salt. Mix then repeat. Finally, drizzle a bit of sweet chili sauce onto the meat and mix again. Use a spoon to scoop out small amounts (1 oz) of meat to form into a meatball. Repeat until the meat is gone, after 16 meatballs. Place the meatballs on a foil lined baking sheet. By now, the oven is hot, place the meatballs in the oven and set a timer for 20 minutes.
3. Meanwhile, the water has come to a boil, pour broccoli into the water. Allow to continue to cook on high heat.
4. Place a pan coated with cooking spray over high heat to warm the pan. When the pan is hot, pour in the pot stickers. Stir continuously while for 2 minutes.

After 2 minutes, add enough water to the pan to cover the bottom. Cover the pan. Reduce the heat to low and allow to steam for 5 minutes.

5. Finally, remove the broccoli from the stove. Drain and cover to keep warm.

Your active cooking is done!
Let your appliances do the rest!

When the timer alarms, remove the meatballs from the oven. Serve meal with a side of sweet chili sauce for dipping.

---------- Figure Friendly Meal Notes ----------

This Figure Friendly Meal includes starch for the satisfaction factor. If you're more satisfied by fat, skip the pot stickers. Add butter or sesame oil to your broccoli instead.

Korean Beef Bowl

Active Cooking:10 min | Total Cooking: 13 min | Serves 4

Appliances: Pressure Cooker

Ingredients:

- 1 cup rice
- 2 cups water
- 1 lb. lean ground meat (turkey, chicken, or beef)

- 4 shakes season salt
- 10 shakes garlic powder
- 10 shakes umami seasoning
- ¼ cup soy sauce
- ¼ cup brown sugar
- ½ lime
- 2 spoonsful vinegar, rice wine
- 5 shakes ground ginger
- 1 lb. bag broccoli florets, frozen

Directions:

1. Put a medium pot half full of water on the stove over high heat. Place the rice and water inside of the pressure cooker and set for 4 minutes on the manual setting.
2. Season the ground meat with 2 shakes of season salt as well as 5 shakes each of garlic and umami seasoning. Mix and repeat.
3. In a bowl, whisk together the soy sauce, brown sugar, juice of a lime, rice wine vinegar, and ginger.
4. Meanwhile, the water has come to a boil. Pour the broccoli into the pot and continue to cook on high heat.
5. Place an empty pan over high heat to warm. When the pan is hot, crumble the ground meat into the pan. Stir continuously to prevent burning or sticking until the meat browns, 7 minutes.
6. When about half of the meat is browned, remove the broccoli from the stove. Drain the water and cover to keep warm.
7. When the meat browns, pour the soy sauce mixture into the pan. Stir to combine ingredients. Then,

cover and reduce heat to low. Allow to simmer for 3 minutes.

Your active cooking is done!
Let your appliances do the rest.

When the meat is done simmering, remove from the stove. Place one-fourth of each ingredient in a bowl to create one serving. Layer in this order: rice, meat, broccoli.

---------- *Figure Friendly Meal Notes* ----------

This Figure Friendly Meal includes starch for the satisfaction factor. If you are more satisfied by fat, skip the rice. Serve over cauliflower rice instead and enjoy some dark chocolate for dessert.

Lettuce Wraps

Active Cooking: 10 min | Total Cooking: 13 min | Serves 4

Appliances: None

Ingredients:

- 8 iceberg or butter lettuce leaves
- ¼ cup soy sauce
- ¼ cup brown sugar
- ½ lime
- 2 spoonsful vinegar, rice wine
- 5 shakes ground ginger

- 1 lb. lean ground meat (turkey, chicken, or beef)
- 4 shakes season salt
- 10 shakes garlic powder
- 10 shakes umami seasoning

Directions:

1. Rinse the lettuce leaves. Place on paper towels in a single layer to drain.
2. In a bowl, whisk together the soy sauce, brown sugar, ginger, lime, and rice wine vinegar.
3. Season the ground meat with 2 shakes of season salt as well as 5 shakes each of garlic powder and umami seasoning. Mix and repeat.
4. Place an empty pan over high heat until it is warm. When the pan is hot, crumble the meat into the pan. Stir continuously to avoid sticking or burning. Continue stirring until meat is browned, 7 minutes. Pour the soy sauce mixture into the meat. Reduce heat to low. Cover and simmer for 3 minutes.

Your active cooking is done!
Let your appliances do the rest!

When the meat is done, divide equally onto the lettuce leaves.

---------- *Figure Friendly Meal Notes* ----------

This Figure Friendly Meal doesn't include a significant portion of either satisfaction factor, fat or starch. If you're more satisfied by starch, add some rice to your lettuce wraps. If you're more satisfied by fat, add sliced almonds to your lettuce wraps.

Meatloaf & Roasted Potatoes with Asparagus

Active Cooking: 7 min | Total Cooking: 47 min | Serves 4

Appliances: Oven

Ingredients:

- 8 small red potatoes
- 13 shakes season salt, divided
- 13 shakes garlic powder, divided
- 1 bunch asparagus
- 1 lb. lean ground meat (turkey, chicken, or beef)
- 10 shakes oregano
- 10 shakes basil
- 1 egg
- ½ cup marinara sauce, divided

Directions:

1. Preheat the oven to 350F.
2. While rinsing with water, rub the potatoes vigorously to remove dirt. Cut the potatoes into ½-inch slices. Place them on a foil lined baking sheet that is coated with cooking spray. Season the potatoes with 3 shakes each of season salt and garlic powder and toss. Coat the exposed side of the potatoes with cooking spray.
3. Rinse the asparagus and place on the same foil lined baking sheet as the potatoes using a foil divider to keep them separate.
4. Season the ground meat with 5 shakes each of season salt, garlic powder, oregano, and basil. Mix and repeat. Crack the egg and add it to the meat mixture along with half of the marinara sauce. Mix

well to combine ingredients. Place the meat mixture into a loaf style baking dish and smooth the top.

5. Place the meatloaf, potatoes, and asparagus in the oven. Set a timer for 25 minutes.

Your active cooking is done!
Let your appliances do the rest!

After 25 minutes, remove the asparagus, potatoes, and meatloaf from the oven. Cover the potatoes and asparagus with foil to keep warm. Pour remaining marinara sauce on top of the meatloaf, and place into the oven for an additional 15 minutes before removing for the final time.

---------- *Figure Friendly Meal Notes* ----------

This Figure Friendly Meal includes starch for the satisfaction factor. If you're more satisfied by fat, skip the potatoes, and drizzle olive oil over your asparagus.

Sweet Basil Spaghetti & Simple Salad

Active Cooking: 11 min | Total Cooking: 17 min | Serves 4

Appliances: Pressure Cooker

Ingredients:

- 2 tomatoes, sliced
- 2 bags (10 oz) shredded iceberg lettuce
- 1 lb. lean ground meat (turkey, chicken, or beef)

- 10 shakes season salt
- 10 shakes garlic powder
- 10 shakes oregano
- 10 shakes basil
- 2 jars sweet basil marinara sauce
- ½ box (16 oz) spaghetti
- Italian Dressing, to taste

Directions:

1. Set the pressure cooker to the sauté setting.
2. Rinse the tomatoes and slice into ½-inch thick pieces. Place the tomatoes and lettuce in a large salad bowl. Toss to combine ingredients.
3. Season the ground meat with 5 shakes each of season salt, garlic powder, oregano, and basil. Mix and repeat. Crumble the meat into the pressure cooker while constantly stirring until the meat is browned, 7 minutes.
4. When the meat is browned, pour the marinara sauce into the pot. Then, break the pasta noodles in half and add to the pot, completely submerging them into the liquid. Cover the pot and set for 6 minutes on the manual setting.

Your active cooking is done!
Let your appliances do the rest!

When the timer alarms, press cancel on your pressure cooker to stop the cooking process. Serve the salad with the dressing on the side.

---------- *Figure Friendly Meal Notes* ----------

This Figure Friendly Meal includes starch for the satisfaction factor. As such, use the salad dressing sparingly. If you're more satisfied by fat, skip the spaghetti. Replace the spaghetti with spiralized zucchini or whole green beans and use the dressing liberally.

Italian Sausage & Peppers with Rice

Active Cooking: 10 min | Total Cooking: 15 min | Serves 4

Appliances: Pressure Cooker

Ingredients:

- 1 cup rice
- 2 cups water
- ½ onion, sliced
- 1 lb. Italian chicken sausage, lean
- 1 bag (16 oz) sliced mixed bell peppers (red, green, yellow, or orange)
- 1 jar (16 oz) sweet tomato basil marina sauce
- 10 shakes basil
- 10 shakes season salt
- 6 shakes black pepper

Directions:

1. Pour the rice and water into the pressure cooker. Set for 4 minutes on the manual setting.

2. Slice one half of an onion into medium slices and slice the sausage into ½-inch pieces.
3. Spray a pan with cooking spray and place the pan over high heat to warm.
4. When the pan is hot, add the peppers and onions and sauté until they soften, 3 minutes. Remove vegetables from the pan.
5. Spray the pan with cooking spray again then place the sausage in the pan. Brown the sausage in the pan while stirring often to prevent burning and sticking. In 5 minutes, add the onions and peppers to the pan. Then, add marinara sauce as well as 10 shakes each of basil and season salt, and 6 shakes of black pepper. Stir to combine ingredients. Reduce heat to low to simmer. Set a timer for 5 minutes.

Your active cooking is done!
Let your appliances do the rest!

When the timer alarms, remove the sausage and peppers from the stove.

---------- *Figure Friendly Meal Notes* ----------

This Figure Friendly Meal includes starch for the satisfaction factor. If you're more satisfied by fat, skip the rice. Replace the rice with cauliflower rice. Then, either use a higher fat sausage or enjoy some dark chocolate.

Mediterranean Meatballs & Rice
with Green Beans

Active Cooking: 7 min | Total Cooking: 52 min | Serves 4

Appliances: Oven

Ingredients:

- 1 cup rice
- 2 cups water
- 1 lb. lean ground meat (turkey, chicken, or beef)
- 8 shakes sea salt
- 6 shakes onion powder
- 10 shakes garlic powder
- 10 shakes oregano
- 10 shakes cumin
- 1 lb. whole green beans, frozen

Directions:

1. Preheat the oven to 350F. Place a medium pot half full of water over high heat to bring to a boil. Add the rice and water to the pressure cooker and set for 4 minutes on the manual setting.
2. Season the ground meat with 4 shakes of sea salt, 3 shakes of onion powder and 5 shakes each of garlic powder, cumin, and oregano. Mix and repeat. Use a spoon to spoon out small portions of meat (about 1 oz) to form into a meatball. Roll the meatball, and continue until all the meat is gone, 16 meatballs. Place meatballs onto a foil lined baking sheet and place them in the oven. Set a timer for 20 minutes.

3. Meanwhile, the water has come to a boil, pour the green beans into the pot. Set a timer for 5 minutes.

**Your active cooking is done!
Let your appliances do the rest!**

When the timer alarms, drain the green beans and cover to keep warm. When the second timer alarms, remove the meatballs from the oven.

---------- *Figure Friendly Meal Notes* ----------

This Figure Friendly Meal includes starch for the satisfaction factor. If you're more satisfied by fat, skip the rice, and drizzle olive oil over your green beans.

Nachos

Active Cooking: 10 min | Total Cooking: 15 min | Serves 4

Appliances: Oven

Ingredients:

- 12 small (6-inch) tortillas, corn
- sea salt, to taste
- 1 lb. lean ground meat (turkey, chicken, or beef)
- 6 shakes season salt
- 1 package taco seasoning
- 1 can (14.4 oz) Rotel
- 1 bag (10 oz) shredded romaine lettuce

- ½ cup cheese, shredded (or break 2 slices into small pieces)
- 1 jar (16 oz) salsa

Directions:

1. Preheat the oven to 350F.
2. Stack tortillas and cut them in half, then in quarters, then in eights. Place the tortillas on a foil lined baking sheet coated with cooking spray. Spray the exposed side with cooking spray. Sprinkle salt over tortillas.
3. Season the ground meat with 3 shakes of season salt. Mix and repeat.
4. Place an empty pan over high heat to warm. When the pan is hot, crumble the meat into the pan. Stir continuously to avoid burning or sticking. Continue until the meat is brown, 7 minutes. When the meat is brown, pour taco seasoning and Rotel into the meat. Stir to combine ingredients. Reduce heat to low and allow to simmer for 5 minutes.
5. Next, place the tortilla chips in the oven, and set a timer for 5 minutes.

Your active cooking is done!
Let your appliances do the rest!

When the timer alarms, remove chips from the oven and meat from the stove. Place one fourth of the chips and meat on each plate. Then, allow each diner to customize their own plate of nachos using the lettuce, cheese, and salsa.

---------- *Figure Friendly Meal Notes* ----------

This Figure Friendly Meal includes starch for the satisfaction factor. If you're more satisfied by fat, use low-carb tortillas, and top your nachos with cheese, sour cream, or guacamole.

Tacos & Cabbage Salad

Active Cooking: 10 min | Total Cooking: 13 min | Serves 4

Appliances: Oven

Ingredients:

- 4 tortillas (8-inch), flour
- 1 lb. lean ground meat (turkey, chicken, or beef)
- 10 shakes season salt
- 10 shakes garlic powder
- 2 spoonsful cumin
- 2 spoonsful chili powder
- 1 spoonful garlic powder
- 2 spoonsful paprika
- 1 spoonful oregano
- 1 spoonful onion powder
- ½ cup water
- 1 bag (10 oz) shredded cabbage
- ½ bag (10 oz) matchstick carrots
- 2 tomatoes, sliced

Directions:

1. Preheat oven to 350F.
2. Place 4 flour tortillas on a foil lined baking sheet coated with cooking spray.
3. Place an empty pan over high heat to warm.
4. Season the ground meat with 5 shakes each of season salt and garlic powder. Mix and repeat.
5. By now, the pan is warm. Crumble the ground meat into the pan and stir continuously until brown, 7 minutes. Add the specified number of spoonsful of cumin, chili powder, garlic powder, paprika, oregano, and onion powder to the pan along with ½ cup of water. Stir to combine ingredients. Reduce heat to low. Cover and simmer for 3 minutes.
6. Place tortillas in the oven.
7. While the meat is simmering, mix cabbage, carrots, and tomatoes in a bowl. Drizzle with a low-fat dressing of your choice

Your active cooking is done!
Let your appliances do the rest!

When the timer alarms, remove the tortillas from the oven and the meat from the stove.

---------- *Figure Friendly Meal Notes* ----------

This Figure Friendly Meal includes starch for the satisfaction factor. If you're more satisfied by fat, use low-carb tortillas, and top your tacos with cheese, sour cream, or guacamole.

Bunless Burger & Fries with Broccoli Slaw

Active Cooking: 4 min | Total Cooking: 16 min | Serves 4

Appliances: Indoor Grill, Oven

Ingredients:

- 1 lb. French fries, frozen (all-natural brand)
- 4 lean burger patties (turkey, chicken, or beef)
- 6 shakes season salt
- 6 shakes garlic powder
- 4 shakes black pepper
- 1 bag (10 oz) Broccoli & Kale Slaw Kit

Directions:

1. Preheat the oven to 425F. Preheat the indoor grill to HIGH.
2. Place the fries on a foil lined baking sheet coated with cooking spray.
3. Season the burger patties with 3 shakes each of season salt and garlic powder as well as 2 shakes of black pepper on each side. Place the burgers on the indoor grill and cook for 8 minutes.
4. Place the fries in the oven and bake until golden brown, 12 minutes.
5. While the burgers and fries are cooking, pour the contents of the slaw kit into a bowl and toss to combine ingredients.

**Your active cooking is done!
Let your appliances do the rest!**

When the timer alarms, remove the burger and fries from the grill and oven. Serve immediately.

---------- *Figure Friendly Meal Notes* ----------

This Figure Friendly Meal includes starch for the satisfaction factor. If you're more satisfied by fat, skip the French fries, and add cheese or avocado slices to your burger.

Concita's Kicking Chili

Active Cooking: 10 min | Total Cooking: 10 min | Serves 4

Appliances: None

Ingredients:

- 1 lb. lean ground meat (turkey, chicken, or beef)
- 6 shakes sea salt
- 6 shakes black pepper
- 6 shakes garlic powder
- 1 can (14.4 oz) kidney beans
- 1 can (14.4 oz) Rotel (replace with diced tomatoes for a milder taste)
- 1 can (14.4 oz) tomato sauce
- 1 packet chili seasoning
- 3 dashes hot sauce (eliminate for a milder taste)

Directions:

1. Season ground meat with 3 shakes each of sea salt, black pepper, and garlic powder. Mix and repeat. Place a large pot coated with cooking spray over high heat to warm. When the pot is hot, crumble ground meat into the pot. Stir continuously until meat is brown, 7 minutes.
2. When the meat is brown, add kidney beans, Rotel, tomato sauce, chili seasoning, and hot sauce to the pot. Stir to combine ingredients. Reduce heat to low. Cover and allow to simmer for 10 minutes.

Your active cooking is done!
Let your appliance do the rest!

When the chili is done, keep covered until you're ready to eat.

---------- *Figure Friendly Meal Notes* ----------

This Figure Friendly Meal includes a small amount of starch. If you're most satisfied by starch, enjoy chili with multi-grain crackers. If you're more satisfied by fat, use half the specified amount of kidney beans. Then, top chili with cheese or avocado slices.

Sweet Potato Chili Boats & Simple Salad

Active Cooking: 10 min | Total Cooking: 55 min | Serves 4

Appliances: Oven

Ingredients:

- 4 medium sweet potatoes
- 1 lb. lean ground meat (turkey, chicken, or beef)
- 6 shakes sea salt
- 6 shakes black pepper
- 6 shakes garlic powder
- 1 can (16 oz) kidney beans
- 1 can (16 0z) tomatoes, diced
- 1 can (16 oz) tomato sauce
- 1 packet chili seasoning
- 2 tomatoes, sliced
- 1 bag (10 oz) shredded romaine lettuce

Directions:

1. Preheat oven to 350 degrees.
2. While rinsing with water, rub the sweet potatoes vigorously to remove dirt. Place on a foil lined baking sheet and use a fork to poke holes in the skin.
3. Season ground meat with 3 shakes each of sea salt, black pepper, and garlic powder. Mix and repeat. Place a large pot coated with cooking spray over high heat to warm. When the pot is hot, crumble ground meat into the pot. Stir continuously until meat is brown, 7 minutes.
4. By now, the oven is hot. Place the potatoes in the oven. Set a timer for 45 minutes.

5. When the meat is brown, add kidney beans, tomatoes, tomato sauce and chili seasoning to the pot. Stir to combine ingredients. Reduce heat to low. Cover and allow to simmer. Set timer for 10 minutes.
6. While the meat simmers, combine lettuce and tomatoes in a large salad bowl. Toss to combine.

Your active cooking is done!
Let your appliances do the rest!

When the timer alarms, remove chili from the stove. Leave covered. When the second timer alarms, remove sweet potatoes from the stove. Cut the potatoes open with one lengthwise cut and place one fourth of the chili mix on top. Serve with salad and low-fat dressing of your choice on the side.

---------- *Figure Friendly Meal Notes* ----------

This Figure Friendly Meal includes starch for the satisfaction factor. If you're most satisfied by fat, skip the sweet potato. Use half the specified amount of kidney beans. Then, top chili with cheese or avocado slices.

Chapter 5

FISH & SEAFOOD

- Fried Catfish & Yams with Kale
- Cajun Shrimp & Rice with Green Beans
- Asian Honey Glazed Salmon & Rice with Broccolini
- Crab House Shrimp & Rice with Broccolini
- Cajun Salmon & Penne with Spinach
- Fish & Chips with Kale Salad
- Lemon Pepper Salmon & Roasted Potatoes with Garlic Parmesan Asparagus
- Lemon Herb Red Snapper & Rice with Asparagus
- Lemon Garlic Shrimp & Linguini with Spinach
- Lemon Pepper Salmon & Rice with Broccolini
- Blackened Catfish & Corn with Green Beans
- Herb Roasted Cod & Rice with Spinach

Fried Catfish & Yams with Kale

Active Cooking: 10 min | Total Cooking: 55 min | Serves 4

Appliances: Oven, Air Fryer

Ingredients:

- 4 medium yams
- 4 catfish fillets (4 ounces each)
- 20 shakes season salt, divided
- 10 shakes garlic powder
- 6 shakes black pepper
- 1 egg
- 1 cup milk
- ½ package (9 oz) Fish Fry
- 1 bag (16 oz) kale, washed and shredded
- 10 shakes onion powder

Directions:

1. Preheat air fryer to 400F. Preheat oven to 350F.
2. While rinsing with water, rub the yams vigorously to remove dirt. Place them on a foil lined baking sheet. Poke the yams with a fork in several places.
3. Rinse catfish fillets with water. Season catfish with 5 shakes each of season salt and garlic powder as well as 3 shakes of black pepper on each side. Crack the egg in a bowl and beat it. Add the milk and mix it again. Place the Fish Fry on a plate and spread it out evenly.
4. Dip each fillet, one at a time, into the egg and milk mixture then immediately press it into the Fish Fry to coat. Next, press the other side into the Fish Fry

to coat. Place the coated fillet on a plate. Continue until all the pieces are coated.

5. By now, the oven is hot. Place the yams in the oven and set a timer for 45 minutes.

6. By now, the air fryer is hot. Spray the inside with cooking spray. Then, place the fish in the fryer. Spray cooking spray on the exposed side of the fish. Finally, close the fryer and set for 10 minutes.

7. While the fish and yams are cooking, heat a pan coated with cooking spray. When the pan is hot, add the kale and stir continuously until the kale softens, 4 minutes. Add enough water to cover the bottom of the pan. Add 10 shakes each of season salt and onion powder and stir. Cover and reduce heat to low. Set a timer for 10 minutes.

Your active cooking is done!
Let your appliances do the rest!

When the fish is done, remove it from the air fryer. Cover with foil to keep warm. When the timer alarms, keep covered and remove kale from heat. When the final timer alarms, remove yams from the oven. There should be brown syrup running out of them. This is a sign that they are done and sweet.

---------- *Figure Friendly Meal Notes* ----------

This Figure Friendly Meal includes starch for the satisfaction factor. If you are more satisfied by fat, skip the yam. Then, enjoy some dark chocolate for dessert.

Cajun Shrimp & Rice with Green Beans

Active Cooking: 10 min | Total Cooking: 13 min | Serves 4

Appliances: Pressure Cooker

Ingredients:

- 1 cup rice
- 2 cups water
- 1 lb. shrimp, deveined
- 10 shakes Cajun seasoning
- ½ onion, chopped
- 1 lb. bell peppers, frozen
- 1 jar (16 oz) marinara sauce
- 5 dashes hot sauce
- 1 bag (16 oz) whole green beans, frozen

Directions:

1. Place a pot half full of water over high heat to bring to a boil. Place the rice and water in the pressure cooker. Set for 4 minutes on the manual setting.
2. Rinse shrimp in water then drain. Season with 5 shakes of Cajun seasoning. Stir and repeat.
3. Place large pan coated with cooking spray over high heat to warm the pan. When the pan is hot, add onion and bell peppers. Stir continuously until the vegetables soften, 4 minutes.
4. Meanwhile, the water has come to a boil. Pour the green beans into the pot. Continue to cook over high heat.
5. Add shrimp to the pan stirring continuously until the shrimp turn pink, 3 minutes. Add marinara sauce and hot sauce to the pot and stir to combine

ingredients. Reduce the heat to low, cover, and set timer for 3 minutes.

6. Remove the green beans from the stove. Drain and keep covered.

Your active cooking is done!
Let your appliances do the rest!

When the timer alarms, turn off the shrimp and remove from heat.

---------- *Figure Friendly Meal Notes* ----------

This Figure Friendly Meal includes starch for the satisfaction factor. If you are more satisfied by fat, skip the rice. Then, drizzle olive oil over your green beans.

Asian Honey Glazed Salmon & Rice

with Broccoli

Active Cooking: 4 min | Total Cooking: 24 min | Serves 4

Appliances: Oven, Pressure Cooker

Ingredients:

- ½ cup rice
- 1 cup water
- 3 spoonsful honey
- ¼ cup soy sauce

- 5 shakes ground ginger
- 4 medium salmon fillets (4 oz each)
- 5 shakes sea salt
- 5 shakes garlic powder
- 5 shakes umami seasoning
- 1 bag (16 oz) broccoli, frozen

Directions:

1. Preheat the oven to 350F. Place rice and water into the pressure cooker. Set for 4 minutes on manual setting. Place medium pot half filled with water on the stove over high heat to bring to a boil.
2. In a bowl, whisk together the honey, soy sauce, and ginger.
3. Rinse the salmon with water and season with 5 shakes each of salt, garlic powder, and umami seasoning. Place the salmon on a foil lined baking sheet. Then, pour honey and soy mixture over the fillets.
4. Meanwhile, the water has come to a boil. Pour the broccoli in the water and continue to cook on high heat. Set a timer for 4 minutes.
5. When the oven is heated, place the salmon in the oven for 20 minutes.

Your active cooking is done!
Let your appliances do the rest!

When the timer alarms, drain the broccoli and cover to keep warm. When the salmon is done, remove from the oven.

---------- *Figure Friendly Meal Notes* ----------

This Figure Friendly Meal includes fat for the satisfaction factor. There is also a small portion of starch. If you find that you are following the Figure Friendly Meal guidelines, but not getting results, consider eliminating the rice from this meal altogether.

Crab House Shrimp & Rice with Broccolini

Active Cooking: 10 min | Total Cooking: 10 min | Serves 4

Appliances: Pressure Cooker

Ingredients:

- 1 cup rice
- 2 cups water
- 1 pat butter (1/8" thick)
- 1 lb. shrimp, deveined
- 8 shakes O'Bay seasoning
- 1 spoonful garlic, minced
- 1 bunch broccolini

Directions:

1. Place the rice and water in a pressure cooker. Set for 4 minutes on manual setting. Place butter in a pan over high heat to melt the butter.

2. Rinse the shrimp and drain excess water. Season the shrimp with 4 shakes of O'Bay seasoning. Mix and repeat.

3. Meanwhile, the butter has melted. Add garlic to the hot butter and continue stirring until the garlic is fragrant, 1 minute. Add the shrimp to the pot and continue cooking. Stir continuously until the shrimp are pink, 3 minutes. Remove from heat and cover to keep warm.

4. Place a pan coated with cooking spray over high heat to warm the pan. When the pan is hot, add the broccolini and cook while stirring often until it is soft, 3 minutes.

Your active cooking is done!

Your meal is ready to be served.

---------- *Figure Friendly Meal Notes* ----------

This Figure Friendly Meal includes starch for the satisfaction factor. If you are more satisfied by fat, skip the yam. Then, drizzle olive oil over the broccolini.

Cajun Salmon & Penne with Spinach

Active Cooking: 7 min | Total Cooking: 20 min | Serves 4

Appliances: Indoor Grill

Ingredients:

- 4 salmon fillets (4 oz each)
- 6 shakes Cajun seasoning
- 6 shakes garlic powder
- ¼ box (13.25 oz) penne pasta
- 1 lb. baby spinach, pre-washed
- ½ jar (16 oz) marinara sauce
- 2 spoonsful basil
- 2 spoonsful oregano
- 1 spoonful lemon pepper
- 1 spoonful garlic
- 1 spoonful sea salt

Directions:

1. Preheat indoor grill to MAX. Place a medium pot half full of water over high heat.
2. Rinse the salmon and season with 6 shakes each of Cajun seasoning and garlic powder.
3. Meanwhile, the water has come to a boil. Pour penne into the pot. Spray cooking spray into the water to prevent sticking Set a timer for 13 minutes.
4. Place a pan coated with cooking over high heat to warm. When the pan is hot, add the spinach. Stir continuously until spinach wilts, 3 minutes. Remove from heat and cover to keep warm.
5. By now the grill is hot. Coat with cooking spray. Place the salmon in the grill and set to 7 minutes.

Your active cooking is done!
Let your appliances do the rest!

When the timer alarms, remove the salmon from the grill and cover to keep warm. When the second timer alarms, drain the penne. Add marinara, basil, oregano, lemon pepper, garlic, and sea salt to the penne. Stir to combine. Cover and allow to sit on the stove over low heat for an additionally 3 minutes.

---------- *Figure Friendly Meal Notes* ----------

This Figure Friendly Meal includes fat for the satisfaction factor. There is also a small portion of starch. If you find that you are following the Figure Friendly Meal guidelines, but not getting results, consider eliminating the pasta from this meal altogether.

Fish & Chips with Kale Salad

Active Cooking: 7 min | Total Cooking: 19 min | Serves 4

Appliances: Air Fryer

Ingredients:

- Sweet Kale Salad Kit
- 4 cod fillets (4 oz each)
- 1 bag (16 oz) French fries, frozen
- 10 shakes sea salt
- 6 shakes black pepper
- 1 egg
- 1 cup milk
- ½ package (9 oz) Fish Fry

Directions:

1. Preheat the air fryer to 400F.
2. Pour all the ingredients (only half of the seeds provided) from the salad kit into a bowl. Toss to combine ingredients.
3. Rinse the cod and season with 5 shakes of salt as well as 3 shakes of black pepper on each side. Crack the egg and beat it. Then, add the milk and mix to combine ingredients. Dip each piece of fish, one at a time, in the egg and milk mixture. Then, press into fish fry to coat. Press the other side into the fish fry to coat. Finally place the coated fillets on a plate.
4. By now, the air fryer is hot. Coat the inside with cooking spray. Place the fish and fries into the air fryer. Spray the exposed side of the fish and fries with cooking spray. Set for the timer for 12 minutes.

Your active cooking is done!
Let your appliances do the rest!

When the fish and fries are done, remove them from the air fryer. Serve immediately.

---------- *Figure Friendly Meal Notes* ----------

This Figure Friendly Meal includes starch for the satisfaction factor. If you are more satisfied by fat, skip the fries. Then, use the entire portion of dressing provided with the salad.

Lemon Pepper Salmon & Roasted Potatoes with Garlic Parmesan Asparagus

Active Cooking: 4 min | Total Cooking: 30 min | Serves 4

Appliances: Oven

Ingredients:

- 1 bunch asparagus
- 4 small red potatoes
- 4 salmon fillets (4 oz each)
- 6 shakes lemon pepper
- 4 shakes salt
- 1 spoonful garlic, minced
- parmesan cheese, to taste

Directions:

1. Preheat the oven to 350F.
2. Rinse the asparagus and the potatoes with water. Be sure to rub the potatoes vigorously while rinsing to remove dirt. Cut the potatoes into ½-inch slices (about 4 per potato). Place the potatoes and asparagus on a foil lined baking sheet covered with cooking spray. Use a foil divider to separate the asparagus from the potatoes.
3. Rinse the salmon fillets and season with 4 shakes of salt as well 6 shakes of lemon pepper. Place the salmon on a foil lined baking sheet covered with cooking spray.
4. By now, the oven is heated. Place the salmon, potatoes and asparagus in the oven. Set a timer for 20 minutes.

Your active cooking is done!
Let your appliances do the rest!

When the timer alarms, remove the asparagus from the oven. Top with minced garlic and parmesan cheese and return to oven. Set a timer for 5 minutes. When the timer alarms for the final time, remove all the food from the oven.

---------- *Figure Friendly Meal Notes* ----------

This Figure Friendly Meal includes fat for the satisfaction factor. There is also a small portion of starch. If you find that you are following the Figure Friendly Meal guidelines, but not getting results, consider eliminating the potatoes from this meal altogether.

Lemon Herb Red Snapper & Rice with Asparagus

Active Cooking: 3 min | Total Cooking: 28 min | Serves 4

Appliances: Oven, Pressure Cooker

Ingredients:

- 1 cup rice
- 2 cups water
- 1 bunch asparagus
- 4 red snapper fillets (4 oz each)
- 6 shakes herbs de provence

- 4 shakes sea salt
- 4 shakes black pepper

Directions:

1. Preheat the oven to 350F. Place the rice and water in the pressure cooker. Set for 4 minutes on manual setting.
2. Rinse the asparagus and place on a foil lined baking sheet covered with cooking spray.
3. Rinse the fish with water. Season with 6 shakes herbs de provence as well as 4 shakes each of salt and black pepper. Place the fish on the same foil lined baking sheet as the asparagus. Be sure to use a foil divider to keep the fish and asparagus separate.
4. Put the fish and the asparagus in the oven. Set a timer for 25 minutes.

Your active cooking is done!
Let your appliance do the rest!

When the timer alarms, remove the snapper and asparagus from the oven.

---------- *Figure Friendly Meal Notes* ----------

This Figure Friendly Meal includes starch for the satisfaction factor. If you are more satisfied by fat, skip the rice. Then, drizzle olive oil over the asparagus.

Lemon Garlic Shrimp & Linguini with Spinach

Active Cooking: 5 min | Total Cooking: 17 min | Serves 4

Appliances: None

Ingredients:

- 1 bag (16 oz) spinach, pre-washed
- ½ box (16 oz) linguini
- 1 lb. shrimp, deveined
- 10 shakes garlic powder
- 10 shakes lemon pepper
- 10 shakes sea salt, divided
- 1 spoonful basil
- 1 spoonful oregano
- parmesan cheese

Directions:

1. Put a medium pot half filled with water on the stove over high heat to bring to a boil.
2. Place a pan coated with cooking spray over high heat to warm. When pan is warm, add spinach. Stir continuously until spinach wilts, 3 minutes. Cover and remove from heat.
3. Meanwhile, the water has come to a boil. Pour linguini in the water and spray cooking spray into the pot to prevent sticking. Set a timer for 12 minutes.
4. Rinse the shrimp and season with 5 shakes each of garlic powder and lemon pepper as well as 2 shakes of salt. Mix and repeat. Place a pan coated with cooking spray over high heat to warm. When the pan is hot, add the shrimp. Stir continuously until the shrimp is pink, 3 minutes.

Your active cooking is done!
Let your appliances do the rest!

When the timer alarms, drain linguini. Add shrimp, basil, oregano and 6 shakes of salt to the pot. Mix to combine ingredients. Serve with parmesan cheese on the side.

---------- *Figure Friendly Meal Notes* ----------

This Figure Friendly Meal includes starch for the satisfaction factor. If you are more satisfied by fat, replace the Linguini with spiralized zucchini. Then, add butter to the spinach.

Lemon Pepper Salmon & Rice with Broccolini

Active Cooking: 5 min | Total Cooking: 12 min | Serves 4

Appliances: Indoor Grill, Pressure Cooker

Ingredients:

- 1 cup rice
- 2 cups water
- 4 salmon fillets (4 oz each)
- 5 shakes season salt
- 5 shakes garlic powder
- 5 shakes lemon pepper
- 1 bunch broccolini

Directions:

1. Preheat the indoor grill to MAX. Place the rice and water in the pressure cooker. Set for 4 minutes on the manual setting.
2. Place a pan coated with cooking spray over high heat to warm the pan. When the pan is hot, add the broccolini. Stir continuously until broccolini is soft, 3 minutes.
3. Rinse the salmon and season with 5 shakes each of salt, garlic powder, and lemon pepper.
4. By now, the grill is heated. Coat with cooking spray. Place the salmon on the grill and set the timer for 7 minutes.

Your active cooking is done!
Let your appliances do the rest!

When the salmon is done, remove from the grill. Serve immediately.

---------- *Figure Friendly Meal Notes* ----------

This Figure Friendly Meal includes fat for the satisfaction factor. There is also a small portion of starch. If you find that you are following the Figure Friendly Meal guidelines, but not getting results, consider eliminating the rice from this meal altogether.

Blackened Catfish & Corn with Green Beans

Active Cooking: 4 min | Total Cooking: 24 min | Serves 4

Appliances: Oven, Microwave

Ingredients:

- 4 catfish fillets (4 oz each)
- 10 shakes blackened seasoning
- 2 ears corn, still in husk
- 1 bag (16 oz) whole green beans, frozen

Directions:

1. Preheat the oven to 375. Place a medium pot half full of water over high heat to bring to a boil.
2. Rinse the fish and season it with 5 shakes of blackening season on each side. Place the fish on a foil lined baking sheet coated with cooking spray.
3. Place the corn in the microwave and set it for 5 minutes.
4. Meanwhile, the water has come to a boil. Pour green beans into the pot.
5. By now, the oven is heated, place catfish in the oven. Set a timer for 20 minutes.

Your active cooking is done!
Let your appliances do the rest!

When the corn is done, leave it in the microwave and remove the green beans from the stove. Drain the green beans and cover to keep warm. When the timer alarms, remove the catfish from the oven and the corn from the microwave. Remove the husk of the corn and serve immediately.

---------- *Figure Friendly Meal Notes* ----------

This Figure Friendly Meal doesn't include a full portion of either satisfaction factor, fat or starch. If you're more satisfied with starch, enjoy with a slice of bread or small dinner roll. If you're more satisfied by fat, add butter to your corn.

Herb Roasted Cod & Rice with Spinach

Active Cooking: 7 min | Total Cooking: 16 min | Serves 4

Appliances: Oven, Pressure Cooker

Ingredients:

- 1 cup rice
- 2 cups water
- 1 lemon, sliced
- 4 cod fillets (4 oz each)
- 10 shakes herbs de provence
- 6 shakes garlic powder
- 4 shakes lemon pepper
- 1 bag (16 oz) baby spinach, pre-washed

Directions:

1. Preheat the oven to 400F. Place the rice and water in the pressure cooker. Set for 4 minutes on manual setting.
2. Rinse a lemon and cut into ½-inch thick slices.
3. Rinse the cod and season with 5 shakes of herbs de provence as well as 3 shakes of garlic powder and 2 shakes of lemon pepper on each side. Place the fish in a foil pouch and place lemon on top of the fish before sealing the pouch. Place the foil pouch on a foil lined baking sheet. Place the fish in the oven and bake for 12 minutes.
4. While the fish is baking, place a pan coated with cooking spray over high heat. When the pan is hot, add spinach. Stir continuously until spinach wilts, 3 minutes. Cover and remove from heat.

Your active cooking is done!
Let your appliances do the rest!

When the timer alarms, remove cod from the oven. Let stand for 3 minutes before serving.

---------- *Figure Friendly Meal Notes* ----------

This Figure Friendly Meal includes starch for the satisfaction factor. If you are more satisfied by fat, skip the rice. Then, drizzle olive oil over your spinach.

Chapter 6

ENTRÉE SALADS

- Southwest Chicken Salad
- Shrimp & Strawberry Salad
- Salmon Spring Salad
- Mandarin Almond Chicken Salad
- Asian Shrimp Salad
- Jerk Chicken & Mango Salad
- Burger Salad
- Simple Taco Salad
- Chicken Apple Walnut Salad
- Chef Salad
- Greek Chicken Salad
- BBQ Chicken Salad
- Sausage Salad

Southwest Chicken Salad

Active Cooking: 5 min | Total Cooking: 18 min | Serves 4

Appliances: Indoor Grill

Ingredients:

- 2 tomatoes, sliced
- 2 stalks scallion, sliced
- ½ cup salsa
- ½ cup Ranch dressing
- 1 spoonful taco seasoning
- 1 lb. chicken tenderloins
- 10 shakes season salt
- 10 shakes cumin
- 10 shakes garlic powder
- 6 shakes chili powder
- 2 bags (10 oz) shredded romaine lettuce
- 1 cup corn, drained

Directions:

1. Preheat the indoor grill to HIGH.
2. Rinse and slice the tomatoes and scallions. Drain the corn.
3. Mix the salsa, salad dressing, and taco seasoning together.
4. Rinse the chicken with water and the juice of a lime. Then, rinse and drain. Season the chicken with 5 shakes each of season salt, cumin, and garlic powder as well as 3 shakes of chili powder on each side.
5. By now, the grill will be hot. Coat the grill with cooking spray. Place the chicken on the grill and set the timer for 12 minutes.

6. While the chicken is cooking, toss the lettuce, scallions, corn, and tomatoes in a large salad bowl.

**Your active cooking is done!
Let your appliances do the rest!**

When the chicken is done, cut it into ½-inch thick pieces and toss the chicken, lettuce mixture, and dressing mixture until the ingredients are combined.

---------- *Figure Friendly Meal Notes* ----------

This Figure Friendly Meal includes fat as the satisfaction factor. If you're more satisfied by starch, add crushed tortilla chips (about 20 chips) to your salad. Then, when making the dressing, replace ¼ cup of the Ranch dressing with ¼ cup of salsa to reduce the fat content of the meal.

Shrimp & Strawberry Salad

Active Cooking: 10 min | Total Cooking: 10 min | Serves 4

Appliances: Salad Chopper

Ingredients:

- 2 bags (10 oz) baby spinach
- 1 cup strawberries, sliced
- 1 lb. shrimp, thawed and cleaned
- 8 shakes sea salt
- 8 shakes black pepper

- ½ cup Raspberry Vinaigrette dressing

Directions:

1. Place spinach in your salad chopper bowl and chop as fine as preferred.
2. Rinse strawberries and slice before adding to the bowl with the spinach.
3. Coat a pan with cooking spray and place over high heat to warm the pan.
4. Rinse the shrimp with water and drain. Season with 4 shakes of each of sea salt and black pepper. Stir to mix and repeat. By now, the pan is hot. Add shrimp to the pan and cook until they turn pink, 4 minutes. Be sure to continue stirring to avoid sticking or burning.
5. Add shrimp and dressing to the spinach mixture and toss to combine ingredients.

Your active cooking is done!

---------- Figure Friendly Meal Notes ----------

This Figure Friendly Meal includes fat as the satisfaction factor. If you're more satisfied by starch, enjoy with multi-grain crackers. Then, use the dressing sparingly or replace it with a low-fat dressing like Honey Mustard dressing to reduce the fat content of the meal.

Salmon Spring Salad

Active Cooking: 5 min | Total Cooking: 12 min | Serves 4

Appliances: Salad Chopper, Indoor Grill

Ingredients:

- 1 cucumber, chopped
- 1 peach, chopped
- ½ red onion, chopped
- 2 bags (10 oz) spring mix greens
- 1 cup cherry tomatoes
- ½ cup Citrus Vinaigrette Dressing
- 4 salmon fillets (4 oz each)
- 6 shakes salt
- 4 shakes black pepper

Directions:

1. Preheat indoor grill to MAX.
2. Rinse cucumber with water. Then, peel with a potato peeler, and chop into fourths. Rinse peach and chop into fourths. Chop ½ an onion in half. Place greens, cucumber, onions, and peaches into your salad chopper bowl and chop as fine as preferred. Then add tomatoes and dressing and toss to combine ingredients.
3. Season salmon with 6 shakes of salt and 4 shakes of black pepper.
4. By now, the grill is hot. Place salmon on the grill, flesh side down, and set for 7 minutes.

Your active cooking is done!
Let your appliances do the rest!

When the salmon is cooked, remove it from the grill and remove skin before serving.

---------- *Figure Friendly Meal Notes* ----------

This Figure Friendly Meal includes fat as the satisfaction factor. If you're more satisfied by starch, enjoy with multi-grain crackers. Then, use only half of the walnuts recommended and use the dressing sparingly or replace it with a low-fat dressing like Honey Mustard dressing to reduce the fat content of the meal.

Mandarin Almond Chicken Salad

Active Cooking: 5 min | Total Cooking: 17 min | Serves 4

Appliances: Indoor Grill

Ingredients:

- 1 lb. chicken tenderloins
- 10 shakes salt
- 10 shakes umami seasoning
- 10 shakes black pepper
- 1 bag (10 oz) shredded cabbage
- 1 bag (10 oz) shredded romaine lettuce
- ½ bag (10 oz) matchstick carrots
- ½ can (16 oz) Mandarin oranges
- 1 scallion, sliced
- ¼ cup almonds, sliced
- ½ cup Honey Mustard Dressing

Directions:

1. Preheat the indoor grill to HIGH.
2. In a large bowl, wash the chicken with water. Then, rinse and drain. Season the chicken with 5 shakes each of salt, umami seasoning, and black pepper on each side.
3. Add the cabbage, romaine lettuce, carrots, Mandarin oranges, scallions, and almonds to a large salad bowl.
4. By now, the grill is hot. Place the chicken in the indoor grill and set to 12 minutes.

**Your active cooking is done!
Let your appliances do the rest!**

When the chicken is done, slice it into ½- inch thick pieces and add to the bowl of salad along with the dressing. Toss to combine ingredients.

---------- Figure Friendly Meal Notes ----------

This Figure Friendly Meal doesn't include a significant source of either satisfaction factor, fat or starch. If you're more satisfied by starch, enjoy with multi-grain crackers. If you're more satisfied with fat, use double the amount of almonds specified above and a higher fat dressing of your choice.

Asian Shrimp Salad

Active Cooking: 10 min | Total Cooking: 10 min | Serves 4

Appliances: Salad Chopper

Ingredients:

- 1 T coconut oil
- 1 lb. shrimp, pre-cooked
- 6 shakes salt
- 6 shakes black pepper
- 1 head green cabbage
- ½ head purple cabbage
- 1 bag (10 oz) matchstick carrots
- 1 cup grape tomatoes
- 1 cup red grapes
- ½ cup Sesame Ginger Dressing

Directions:

1. Place a pan with coconut oil over high heat to melt.
2. Rinse shrimp with water. Drain and season with 3 shakes each of salt and black pepper. Stir to mix then repeat. By now, the oil is melted and hot. Add the shrimp to the pan, and sauté the shrimp for 2-3 minutes, continuously stirring to avoid sticking or burning. Cover and remove from heat.
3. Cut the cabbage into eights. Rinse, drain, and place in the salad chopper bowl and chop as fine as preferred. Add the carrots, grape tomatoes, grapes, dressing, and shrimp to the bowl. Toss to combine ingredients.

Your active cooking is done!

---------- *Figure Friendly Meal Notes* ----------

This Figure Friendly Meal includes fat as the satisfaction factor. If you're more satisfied by starch, enjoy with multi-grain crackers. Then, use cooking spray, instead of coconut oil to sauté the shrimp, and half of the dressing recommended or a low-fat dressing of your choice to reduce fat content of the meal.

Jerk Chicken & Mango Salad

Active Cooking: 5 min | Total Cooking: 17 min | Serves 4

Appliances: Salad Chopper, Indoor Grill

Ingredients:

- 2 bags (10 oz) spring mix greens
- 1 medium mango
- ½ can (16 oz) sweet peas, drained
- 1 lb. chicken tenderloins
- 1 lime
- 10 shakes season salt
- 10 shakes garlic powder
- 1 spoonful jerk seasoning paste
- ½ cup Citrus Vinaigrette dressing

Directions:

1. Preheat the indoor grill to HIGH.

2. Pour the greens into the salad chopper bowl. Remove the pit of the mango and chop it into fourths. Use the salad chopper to chop the greens and mango as fine as preferred. Drain peas and add them to the bowl.

3. In a large bowl, wash the chicken with water and the juice of a lime. Then, rinse and drain. Season the chicken with 5 shakes each of salt and garlic powder on each side. Add the Jerk seasoning paste and stir to distribute evenly. By now, the grill is hot. Coat with cooking spray. Place the chicken on the grill and set for 12 minutes.

Your active cooking is done!
Let your appliances do the rest!

When the chicken is done, cut it into ½-inch thick slices. Add the chicken and dressing to the salad bowl and toss to combine ingredients.

---------- *Figure Friendly Meal Notes* ----------

This Figure Friendly Meal includes fat as the satisfaction factor. If you're more satisfied by starch, enjoy with multi-grain crackers. Then, use only half of the walnuts recommended and use the dressing sparingly or replace it with a low-fat dressing like Honey Mustard dressing to reduce the fat content of the meal.

Burger Salad

Active Cooking: 4 min | Total Cooking: 12 min | Serves 4

Appliances: Indoor Grill

Ingredients:

- 2 bags (10 oz) shredded romaine lettuce
- 1 cup grape tomatoes
- 1 bag (16 oz) matchstick carrots
- ½ cup pickle slices
- 4 turkey burgers patties (4 oz), lean
- 6 shakes season salt
- 6 shakes garlic powder
- 6 shakes black pepper
- ½ cup Honey Mustard Dressing

Directions:

1. Preheat the indoor grill to HIGH.
2. Place lettuce, grape tomatoes, carrots, and pickle slices in a large salad bowl, and toss to combine ingredients.
3. Season the turkey burger patties with 3 shakes each of season salt, garlic powder, and black pepper on each side.
4. By now, the grill is hot. Place the patties on the grill and set to 7 minutes.

Your active cooking is done!
Let your appliances do the rest!

When the burgers are done, chop them into eights. Add the burgers along with the dressing to the salad bowl and toss to combine ingredients.

---------- *Figure Friendly Meal Notes* ----------

This Figure Friendly Meal doesn't include a significant amount of either satisfaction factor, starch or fat. If you're more satisfied by starch, enjoy with a side of baked French fries. If you're more satisfied by fat, add avocado slices to the salad or use a higher fat dressing of your choice.

Simple Taco Salad

Active Cooking: 10 min | Total Cooking: 10 min | Serves 4

Appliances: None

Ingredients:

- 1 lb. ground meat (turkey, chicken, beef)
- 10 shakes season salt
- 10 shakes garlic powder
- 2 spoonsful cumin
- 2 spoonsful chili powder
- 1 spoonful garlic powder
- 2 spoonsful paprika
- 1 spoonful oregano
- 1 spoonful onion powder
- ½ cup water
- 2 tomatoes, chopped

- 2 bags (10 oz) shredded romaine lettuce
- Green Tomatillo Sauce

Directions:

1. Place a large pan over high heat to warm pan.
2. Season the meat with 5 shakes each of season salt and garlic powder. Mix then repeat. Crumble the meat into the pan and continue stirring to avoid sticking or burning until the meat browns, 7 minutes. When the meat browns, dump the spoonsful of cumin, chili powder, garlic powder, paprika, oregano, and onion powder into the meat. Add the water and mix well to combine the ingredients. Reduce the heat to low, cover, and simmer for 4 minutes.
3. While the meat is simmering, rinse the tomatoes with water. Then, dice the tomatoes into medium pieces.
4. Add the tomatoes, lettuce, meat, and green tomatillo sauce to a large salad bowl. Toss to combine.

Your active cooking is done!

---------- Figure Friendly Meal Notes ----------

This Figure Friendly Meal doesn't include a satisfaction factor, starch or fat. If you're more satisfied by starch, enjoy with a serving of tortilla chips, 20 chips. If you're more satisfied by fat, add avocado slices, cheese, or a higher fat dressing of your choice.

Chicken Apple Walnut Salad

Active Cooking: 5 min | Total Cooking: 17 min | Serves 4

Appliances: Indoor Grill

Ingredients:

- 2 medium Gala apples
- 2 bags (10 oz) shredded romaine lettuce
- 1 bag (10 oz) matchstick carrots
- 1 small box raisins
- 4 spoonsful walnuts, pieces
- 1 lb. chicken tenderloins
- 10 shakes salt
- 10 shakes garlic powder
- ½ cup Raspberry Vinaigrette Dressing

Directions:

1. Preheat indoor grill to HIGH.
2. Rinse the apples with water. Core them and cut them into ½-inch slices. Finally add them to a large salad bowl. Add the romaine lettuce, carrots, raisins, and walnuts to the salad bowl. Toss to combine ingredients.
3. In a large bowl, wash the chicken with water. Then, rinse and drain. Season the chicken with 5 shakes each of salt and garlic powder each on each side. By now, the grill is hot. Coat the grill with cooking spray. Place the chicken in the grill and set to 12 minutes.

Your active cooking is done!
Let your appliances do the rest!

When the chicken is done, cut it into ½-inch slices. Add the chicken along with the dressing to the salad bowl. Toss to combine ingredients.

---------- *Figure Friendly Meal Notes* ----------

This Figure Friendly Meal includes fat as the satisfaction factor. If you're more satisfied by starch, enjoy with multi-grain crackers. Then, use only half of the walnuts recommended and use the dressing sparingly or replace it with a low-fat dressing like Honey Mustard dressing to reduce the fat content of the meal.

Chef Salad

Active Cooking: 5 min | Total Cooking: 12 min | Serves 4

Appliances: Salad Chopper

Ingredients:

- 4 eggs, boiled
- 2 cucumbers, chopped
- 2 bags (10 oz) chopped romaine lettuce
- 1 bag (10 oz) matchstick carrots
- 1 package (8 oz) turkey deli meat (all-natural)
- 1 package (8 oz) ham deli meat (all-natural)
- Honey Mustard Dressing, to taste

Directions:

1. Place a medium pot filled with water and 4 eggs over high heat to bring to a boil.
2. Rinse the cucumbers with water then peel them with a potato peeler. Chop into fourths and place in the salad chopper bowl. Use the salad chopper to chop cucumbers as fine as desired. Add the romaine lettuce and carrots to the bowl.
3. Open each package of deli meat. Roll the entire contents of each package into a giant roll. Cut each roll into ¼- inch slices. Then, place the meat in the bowl with the cucumbers and lettuce.

Your active cooking is done!
Let your appliances do the rest!

In 10 minutes, when the eggs are done, rinse them with cold water and peel. Chop into fourths and add them to the salad chopper bowl and toss to combine ingredients. Serve salad with the dressing on the side.

---------- *Figure Friendly Meal Notes* ----------

This Figure Friendly Meal doesn't include a significant amount of either satisfaction factor, starch or fat. If you're more satisfied by starch, enjoy with multi-grain crackers. If you're more satisfied by fat, add avocado slices or cheese.

Greek Chicken Salad

Active Cooking: 7 min | Total Cooking: 20 min | Serves 4

Appliances: Indoor Grill, Salad Chopper

Ingredients:

- 1 bag (16 oz) spring mix greens
- 2 cucumbers
- 2 tomatoes
- 1 lb. chicken tenderloins
- 1 lemon
- 10 shakes sea salt
- 10 shakes garlic powder
- 6 shakes black pepper
- 1 bag (16 oz) shredded romaine lettuce
- 15 green olives
- ½ cup Greek Vinaigrette Dressing

Directions:

1. Preheat the indoor grill to HIGH.
2. Place the Spring Mix lettuce in the salad chopper bowl. Rinse the cucumbers and tomatoes with water. Then, peel the cucumbers with a potato peeler and chop into fourths. Next, chop tomatoes into fourths. Finally, place the cucumbers and tomatoes in the salad chopper bowl. Use the salad chopper to chop the ingredients as fine as preferred.
3. In a large bowl, wash the chicken with water and the juice of a lemon. Then, rinse and drain. Season the chicken with 5 shakes each of salt and garlic powder as well as 3 shakes of black pepper on each side.

4. By now, the indoor grill is heated. Coat with cooking spray. Place the chicken on the grill and set for 12 minutes.
5. While the chicken is cooking, add the romaine lettuce and olives to the salad bowl.

**Your active cooking is done!
Let your appliances do the rest!**

When the chicken is done, slice it into ½-inch thick pieces. Add the chicken and salad dressing to the salad bowl. Toss to combine the ingredients.

---------- *Figure Friendly Meal Notes* ----------

This Figure Friendly Meal includes fat as the satisfaction factor. If you're more satisfied by starch, enjoy with multi-grain crackers. Then, use a low-fat version of the recommended dressing to reduce the fat content of the meal.

BBQ Chicken Salad

Active Cooking: 7 min | Total Cooking: 32 min | Serves 4

Appliances: Salad Chopper, Oven

Ingredients:

- 1 lb. chicken tenderloins
- 10 shakes season salt

- 10 shakes garlic powder
- ½ bottle BBQ sauce
- 2 cucumbers
- 2 tomatoes
- 1 can (16 oz) sweet corn, drained
- 2 bags (16 oz) shredded romaine lettuce
- ¼ cup Ranch Dressing
- ½ cup BBQ sauce

Directions:

1. Preheat the oven to 350F.
2. In a large bowl, wash the chicken with water. Then, rinse and drain. Season with 5 shakes each of season salt and garlic powder on each side of the tenderloins. Place the chicken in a baking dish and cover with ½ bottle BBQ sauce.
3. Rinse the cucumbers and tomatoes with water. Peel the cucumbers with a potato peeler. Then, chop them into fourths and place them in the salad chopper bowl. Next chop the tomatoes into fourths and add them to the salad chopper bowl. Use the salad chopper to chop the ingredients as fine as preferred.
4. By now the oven is heated. Place chicken in the oven and set a timer for 25 minutes.
5. While the chicken is cooking, open the can of corn and drain. Then, add corn to the salad chopper bowl. Add the lettuce to the salad bowl with the rest of the ingredients and toss to combine ingredients.
6. In a separate bowl, mix the ranch dressing with ½ cup BBQ sauce.

Your active cooking is done!
Let your appliances do the rest!

When the timer alarms, remove the chicken from the oven. Cut into ½-inch slices and add to the salad bowl along with the dressing. Toss to combine ingredients.

---------- *Figure Friendly Meal Notes* ----------

This Figure Friendly Meal doesn't include a significant amount of either satisfaction factor, starch or fat. If you're more satisfied by starch, enjoy with multi-grain crackers. If you're more satisfied by fat, add avocado slices or cheese.

Sausage Salad

Active Cooking: 10 min | Total Cooking: 10 min | Serves 4

Appliances: Salad Chopper

Ingredients:

- 1 lb. Italian chicken sausage, lean (about 4)
- 2 cucumbers, chopped
- 2 Gala apples, chopped
- 2 bags (16 oz) shredded romaine lettuce
- ½ cup Honey Mustard Dressing

Directions:

1. Place the sausage in a pan that has been coated with cooking spray. Then, place the pan on a stove over high heat.
2. As the sausage cooks, continue to stir to prevent sticking or burning. After 3 minutes, add enough water to cover the bottom of the pan. Cover the pan and reduce the heat to low. Allow the sausage to continue to cook until the water is gone, 4 minutes.
3. While the sausage is cooking, rinse the cucumbers and apples with water. Use a potato peeler to peel the cucumbers. Chop the cucumbers into fourths and add them to the salad chopper bowl. Core the apples. Chop them into fourths and add them to the salad chopper bowl. Use the salad chopper to chop the cucumbers and apples as fine as preferred. Then, add the romaine lettuce to the mixture.
4. By this time, the sausage should be done. Remove the sausage from the pan and slice the sausage into ½-inch pieces. Then, add the sausage and salad dressing to the bowl. Toss the mixture to combine ingredients.

Your active cooking is done!

---------- Figure Friendly Meal Notes ----------

This Figure Friendly Meal doesn't include a significant portion of either satisfaction factor, fat or starch. If you're more satisfied by starch, enjoy it with some multi-grain crackers. If you're more satisfied by fat, add avocado slices to the salad or use a higher fat dressing of your choice.

PART III

Beyond the Recipes

The recipes included in this book are Figure Friendly and delicious. However, you may want to do a little experimenting on your own. This part of the book will give you the knowledge you need to use the recipes in the book as a springboard to create an infinite number of meals that you can enjoy for years to come.

Chapter 7

HERB & SPICE COMBINATIONS BY CUISINE

You may have noticed that some of our recipes used the same core ingredients. However, we used different spices to create a completely different meal. For example, the main difference between our Asian Meatballs and Mediterranean Meatballs were the spices that we used to season the ground meat. Use the spice combination guide below to go beyond the recipes to create an infinite number of meals that will satisfy your family for years to come. In general, you may have noticed that 10 shakes is the standard amount of each major seasoning in the recipes. You can use more or fewer shakes of any spice to make specific flavors play a prominent role in the taste of your creations.

Asian Food

- ✓ 5-Spice
- ✓ Chili Powder

- ✓ Garlic Powder
- ✓ Ginger, ground
- ✓ Onion Powder
- ✓ Umami

Cajun Food

- ✓ Basil
- ✓ Black Pepper
- ✓ Blackened Seasoning
- ✓ Cajun Seasoning (blend of spices)
- ✓ Cayenne Pepper
- ✓ Cumin, ground
- ✓ Garlic Powder
- ✓ Mustard, dry
- ✓ Onion Powder
- ✓ Oregano
- ✓ Paprika
- ✓ Parsley
- ✓ Thyme

Caribbean Food

- ✓ Allspice
- ✓ Clove
- ✓ Garlic Powder
- ✓ Ginger
- ✓ Jerk Seasoning
- ✓ Nutmeg
- ✓ Paprika
- ✓ Thyme

Italian Food

- ✓ Bay Leaves, dried
- ✓ Basil
- ✓ Garlic Powder
- ✓ Oregano
- ✓ Parsley
- ✓ Rosemary
- ✓ Sage
- ✓ Thyme

Mediterranean Food

- ✓ Allspice
- ✓ Basil
- ✓ Coriander
- ✓ Cumin
- ✓ Dill
- ✓ Garlic Powder
- ✓ Lemon Pepper
- ✓ Oregano
- ✓ Paprika
- ✓ Rosemary
- ✓ Saffron
- ✓ Thyme

Mexican Food

- ✓ Chili Powder
- ✓ Cilantro
- ✓ Cumin
- ✓ Garlic Powder
- ✓ Oregano

Chapter 8

GROCERY & PANTRY STAPLES

Do you prefer to pick your meals day by day instead of creating a plan for the week? If you're more into spontaneity than weekly planning, you'll find this section useful. Here, you'll find a list of the grocery and pantry staples that you'll want to keep on hand to be ready to cook almost any meal in this book on a whim.

Grocery

- ✓ Chicken Breast, boneless and skinless
- ✓ Chicken Roaster, cut in parts
- ✓ Chicken Tenderloins
- ✓ Lean Ground Meat (chicken, turkey, beef)
- ✓ Cod
- ✓ Red Snapper
- ✓ Salmon Fillets
- ✓ Shrimp
- ✓ Asparagus

- ✓ Broccoli
- ✓ Broccolini
- ✓ Cucumbers
- ✓ Green Beans
- ✓ Matchstick Carrots
- ✓ Spinach
- ✓ Shredded Cabbage
- ✓ Shredded Romaine
- ✓ Tomatoes
- ✓ Salad Kits

Pantry

- ✓ Brown Sugar
- ✓ Cooking Spray
- ✓ Olive Oil
- ✓ Coconut Oil
- ✓ Honey Mustard Dressing
- ✓ Marinara Sauce
- ✓ Pasta (linguini, spaghetti, penne)
- ✓ Potatoes (yams, red)
- ✓ Rice
- ✓ Soy Sauce
- ✓ Sweet Chili Sauce
- ✓ Vinaigrette Dressing (Citrus, Greek, Raspberry)
- ✓ Rotel
- ✓ Yellow Thai Curry Sauce

Chapter 9

KITCHEN TOOLS & APPLIANCES

As you learned earlier in this book, the right tools and appliances can dramatically reduce your active cooking time. You don't need to purchase every appliance that hits the market, but a few key appliances can make a big difference. Many of the recipes in this book use the oven, as that's an appliance that I'm confident you have. Below, you'll find the other kitchen tools and appliances that I recommend.

Potato Peeler

This tool is perfect for peeling potatoes, cucumbers, and any other fruit or vegetable with thin skin.

Knives

A set of sharp knives can increase the speed and safety of any slicing or chopping you do during meal prep.

Microwave

The microwave helps you thaw meat in minutes on those days you neglect to thaw the meat in advance. It can also be used to quickly reheat food if there's a delay between cooking and mealtime.

Pressure Cooker

The pressure cooker helps you prepare items in a fraction of the time that it takes using other methods. It is also helpful when you need to thaw meat without a lot of time.

Indoor Grill

The indoor grill helps you create delicious grilled dishes without the hassle of outdoor grills. They are also very helpful when you need to go from frozen to cooked while bypassing the thawing step. While you can't do that with every single item in every meal, I've found them especially useful in this regard when it comes to burgers and chicken tenderloins.

Air Fryer

The air fryer helps you create healthy fried dishes without the extra fat or mess involved in deep frying. While you can oven fry items instead of using an air fryer, I've found that the air fryer creates a finished product that more closely mimics the taste and texture of deep-fried food.

Salad Chopper

The salad chopper helps you create those restaurant style chopped salads without the labor. You'll no longer need to slice and dice ingredients by hand. Instead, you'll chop the ingredients into large chunks then quickly chop them with your chopper. Be sure to use the bowl that comes with the chopper for optimal results and safety.

Slow Cooker

The slow cooker is helpful when you need a meal that you can set and forget. One major advantage to slow cooked meals is the ability to cook all the ingredients together without using multiple dishes. Slow cooked meals are also perfect when you want to prep your meal in the morning and come home to a hot, ready to eat meal.

To get a list of brands that I personally use and recommend for each kitchen tool and appliance, visit concitathomas.com/bookextras. That list will be a living document that I will update as I discover better versions of what I currently have.

Beyond the Book

Our time together here is done. You have been equipped with everything you need in order to get delicious Figure Friendly meals on your table each day- in mere minutes. However, the journey toward feeling and looking your best involves more than meals. Anything you really want to achieve in life should be undergirded with support and accountability. Let me help you with this part too!

Join the Free Support Group
Come meet your other Fierce Friends and get tips and support every day.

concitathomas.com/becomeafiercefriend

Join Coaching Club
Get your monthly workout calendar planned for you and enjoy follow along workout videos (feels like we're training together), new monthly recipes, and monthly challenges to help you build the habits necessary to reach your goals. Try it out for free now.

concitathomas.com/trial

Get 1:1 Coaching from Concita
Have specific questions unique to your circumstances? Want to get specialized strategy made just for you? Book a Coaching Call with Concita today.

concitathomas.com/coaching